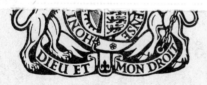

FIT FOR THE FUTURE

Report of the Committee on Child Health Services

Chairman: Emeritus Professor S D M Court, CBE, MD, FRCP, FCST

VOLUME 2

*Presented to Parliament by the Secretary of State for Social Services,
the Secretary of State for Education and Science and the Secretary of
State for Wales by command of Her Majesty*
December 1976

LONDON

HER MAJESTY'S STATIONERY OFFICE

Cmnd. 6684–I

930062

ISBN 0 10 166841 4

STATISTICAL APPENDIX

INTRODUCTION

1. The tables in this appendix are a selection only from the statistical material sought by the Committee at an early stage of its deliberations. Very few of them are new and most of the material in them has already been published elsewhere. However it was felt appropriate to present a balanced statistical appendix both as general background to the report and to support some of the more detailed points made in specific instances.

2. Because a number of different sources of statistics have been used it has not been possible to use the same definitions and classifications throughout. Consequently, age groupings and regional classifications do differ between tables depending on what was available. Most vital and health statistics are available for health authorities but certain general statistics from the Census of Population and the General Household Survey are prepared only for the Standard Statistical Regions of England and these have been quoted to illustrate regional differences where there was no comparable data for health authorities. As many tables as possible have been prepared for England and Wales but for some subjects the most appropriate analysis was available only for Great Britain as a whole: where used these are clearly marked.

3. Reorganisation of Local Government and the National Health Service took place on 1 April 1974. The new Regional and Area Health Authorities then took over functions previously administered by Regional Hospital Boards and Hospital Management Committees (the hospital services), NHS Executive Councils (the general practitioner services) and Local Health Authorities (the community, preventive and school health services). Area Health Authorities' boundaries were made co-terminous with those of the local authorities responsible for social services. The boundaries of Regional Health Authorities are broadly similar to those of the former Regional Hospital Boards but adjusted to take in whole AHA areas. For these reasons, strict comparison on a regional basis is not possible before and after April 1974. Where it seemed useful to make regional comparisons over time the comparison is usually restricted to a period ending in 1973.

4. The tables are presented as follows:

    A. Child population and Births (A.1–16)

    B. Marriage, Family and the Environment (B.1–24)

    C. Infant and child mortality (C.1–12)

    D. Infant and child morbidity (D.1–17)

    E. The use of Health and Personal Social Services by children (E.1–37)

    F. Manpower (F.1–17)

    G. Area profiles (G.1)

Each section is introduced by a short narrative commentary explaining the sequence of the tables and drawing attention to specific trends exhibited by the figures or aspects of the data which need to be fully appreciated in order to avoid misinterpretation. These sections are not intended to provide a full analytic commentary upon the tables. Rather it is hoped that the tables will prove on the whole to be self-explanatory and that the narrative will be an aid to understanding the coverage and the more important patterns and trends.

In compiling the appendix the advice and assistance of members of the staff of the Medical and Population Statistics Divisions of the Office of Population Censuses and Surveys proved invaluable. Without their willing co-operation the task of devising and checking the tables would have been impossible.

A. CHILD POPULATION AND BIRTHS

A.1 Children and young people aged under 20. Estimated home population. Analysis by sex and single years of age, 1961, 1966, 1971, 1973 and 1974.

A.2 Projected population aged under 20. Analysis by age group showing high, central and low variants with migration, 1976, 1981, 1986, 1991, 1996. Great Britain.

A.3 Population aged under 20. Analysis by Regional Health Authority area, showing sex and percentage of total population, 1973 and 1974.

A.4 Children at school. Analysis by type of schooling and showing the percentage remaining at school beyond the statutory leaving age, 1964–1974.

A.5 Population aged under 20. Analysis by sex and age group showing urban/rural aggregates, 1963 and 1973.

A.6 Children with one or both parents born outside the United Kingdom. Analysis by country of origin, 1971 census.

Births

A.7 Live birth rates. Analysis by sex and legitimacy, 1951–1975.

A.8 Births, birth rates and fertility rates. Analysis by Hospital Regions, 1963, 1971 and 1973 (index 1963) and by Regional Health Authority areas, 1974.

A.9 Live births conceived outside marriage. Analysis by Hospital Regions, 1963 and 1973.

A.10 Percentage of children born in NHS hospitals. Analysis by Hospital Regions, 1966 and 1969–1973.

A.11 Births and birth rates. Analysis by age of mother, 1964, 1971, 1973 and 1974.

A.12 High parity births. Analysis by Hospital Regions, 1963, 1971 and 1973.

A.13 Live births. Analysis by birthplace of mother showing numbers and percentage of all live births, 1969–1974.

A.14 Live births. Analysis by birthplace of mother and Regional Health Authority areas, 1974.

2

A.15 Live and stillbirths to females aged under 20. Analysis by single years of age, 1961, 1966, 1971 and 1974.

A.16 Abortions to females aged under 20. Anaylsis by single years of age, 1968–1974.

B.   MARRIAGE, FAMILY AND ENVIRONMENT

B.1 Proportion of women married. Analysis by age, 1911–1974.

B.2 Marriages and marriage rates for men and women, 1951–1974.

B.3 Divorces and divorce rates, 1951–1974.

B.4 Households. Analysis by type of family and number of dependent children, 1971.

B.5 Married couple families with dependent children. Analysis by type and age of head, 1971.

B.6 Estimate of the number of children in one-parent families. Analysis by age, 1971. Great Britain.

Economic Activity

B.7 Percentage of women economically active. Analysis by age and marital status, 1951–1971.

B.8 Wives economically active. Analysis by age and number of dependent children and by age of youngest child, 1971.

B.9 Wives and mothers. Analysis by economic activity and number of dependent children, 1971.

B.10 Children 0–19. Analysis by age and by social class of family head, 1971.

Social Security

B.11 Families receiving Family Allowances. Analysis by size, 1964–1974.

B.12 Families receiving Supplementary Benefit, 1974. Great Britain.

B.13 One-parent families receiving Supplementary Benefit, 1970–1974.

B.14 Families receiving Family Income Supplement, 1974. Great Britain.

B.15 Families receiving Unemployment Benefit, 1968–1974. Great Britain.

B.16 Number of incapacitated males in receipt of Invalidity Benefit and the percentage in receipt of an increase in respect of child dependants with average number of dependent children per father, 1972–1974. Great Britain.

B.17 Chronic sickness among adults over 15. Analysis by age and marital condition, 1973. Great Britain.

B.18 Chronic sickness among adults. Analysis by age and socio-economic group, 1973. Great Britain.

Environment

B.19 Percentage of households lacking or sharing amenities, 1951, 1961, 1966 and 1971.

B.20 Local authority housing. Analysis by storey height and density, 1968–1973.

B.21 People who moved household in previous 12 months, 1973. Great Britain.

B.22 Difference in housing standards between "coloured" and white households, 1971–1973. Great Britain.

B.23 Difference in socio-economic group between "coloured" and white households, 1971–1973. Great Britain.

B.24 Summary statistics of frequency distributions of census indicators, 1971. Great Britain.

C. INFANT AND CHILD MORTALITY

C.1 Death rates for children aged 1–19. Analysis by sex and age group, 1901–1974.

C.2 Stillbirth and infant death rates. Analysis by age, 1906–1974.

C.3 Stillbirths and infant deaths, numbers and rates. Analysis by Hospital Region, 1963, 1966 and 1971–1973.

C.4 International comparisons of infant mortality rates, 1965–1973.

C.5 Live and stillbirths and neonatal deaths. Analysis by birthweight showing numbers and rates, 1954–1974.

C.6 Low weight births. Analysis by Regional Health Authority showing live and stillbirths and death rates, 1974.

C.7 Deaths and death rates of children under 1 year. Analysis by selected causes, 1951, 1961, 1966 and 1971–1974.

C.8 Deaths and death rates of children aged 1–4. Analysis by selected causes, 1951, 1961, 1966 and 1971–1974.

C.9 Deaths and death rates of children aged 5–9. Analysis by selected causes 1951, 1961, 1966 and 1971–1974.

C.10 Deaths and death rates of children aged 10–14. Analysis by selected causes, 1951, 1961, 1966 and 1971–1974.

C.11 Deaths and death rates of young people aged 15–19. Analysis by selected causes, 1951, 1961, 1966 and 1971–1974.

C.12 Number of child deaths and rates per 100,000 per year. Analysis by age and social class, 1959–1963.

D. INFANT AND CHILD MORBIDITY

Congenital Malformations

D.1 Notified congenital malformations showing live and stillborn, 1964–1974.

D.2 Notified congenital malformations. Analysis by site of malformation, sex and type of birth, 1970–1974.

D.3 Notified congenital malformations. Analysis by Standard Region showing rates for selected sites of malformation, 1971–1974.

4

Infectious Diseases

D.4   Infectious diseases notification rates, 1951–1974.

D.5   Infectious diseases notification rates. Analysis by age group, 1974.

Dental Disease

D.6   Percentage of children with dental disease, 1973. (Child Dental Health Survey, 1975).

D.7   Individual dental disease and treatment experience. Analysis by age. (Child Dental Health Survey, 1975).

Hospital

D.8   Special care baby departments. Analysis by diagnosis showing estimated numbers and percentage of discharges from hospital of children aged under one year, 1973.

D.9   Paediatric departments. Discharges and deaths of children under 15. Analysis by diagnostic group showing estimated numbers and percentage of child discharges from all departments, 1973.

D.10   Hospital in-patients aged under 20. Analysis by diagnostic group showing sex and age group, 1973 (index 1968).

D.11   Hospital in-patients aged under 20. Average daily bed rates per million population. Analysis by diagnostic group showing sex and age group, 1973 (index 1968).

D.12   Hospital in-patients aged under 20. Mean duration of stay. Analysis by diagnostic group showing sex and age group, 1973 (index 1968).

D.13   Hospital in-patients aged under 15. Discharge rates. Analysis by sex and Regional Hospital Board area of residence showing selected diagnoses, 1973.

D.14   Venereal disease. New cases. Analysis by sex and age group, 1966–1974.

General Medical Practice

D.15   Children and young people aged under 25 consulting a general medical practitioner. Rates per 1,000 population. Analysis by diagnostic group and age group, 1970–1971.

Attendance Allowance

D.16   Attendance allowances in payment in respect of children and young people aged 2–19. Analysis by sex and Standard Region, 1972 and 1974.

D.17   Attendance allowances in payment in respect of children and young people aged 2–19. Analysis by main cause of helplessness showing age group and sex, 1974.

E. THE USE OF HEALTH AND PERSONAL SOCIAL SERVICES BY CHILDREN

Preventive Health and Community Care

E.1 Number of premises in use as maternity and child health centres. Analysis by type of premises, 1964 and 1971–1974.

E.2 Number of children attending and number of sessions held at child health centres, 1964 and 1971–1974.

E.3 Percentage of children vaccinated and immunised for certain diseases. Analysis by Regional Hospital Board areas, 1971–1973.

E.4 Number of children consulting general medical practitioners for all reasons and those immunised, 1970–1971.

E.5 Children consulting general medical practitioners. Consultations per person, percentage distribution and rate per thousand by site of consultation, 1971–1973.

E.6 Children consulting general medical practitioners. Analysis by sex, age group and Standard Region, 1971–1972.

E.7 Child referrals from general medical practitioners to another agency, 1970–1971.

E.8 Community health dental services for children under 5, 1966–1974.

E.9 School Health Service. Analysis by number of medical inspections and cause, 1964–1974.

Personal Social Services

E.10 Children's day care facilities, 1972–1975.

E.11 Children in care of local authorities at 31 March 1972–1975.

E.12 Circumstances in which children came into care of local authorities (excluding remand and interim orders), 1972–1975.

E.13 Numbers aged under 16 on the registers for the general classes of handicap, deaf and blind, 1964, 1970, 1974 and 1975.

Non-Psychiatric Hospitals

E.14 Discharge rates for children aged 0–19. Analysis by sex and age group, 1960–1973 (index 1964).

E.15 Average beds occupied daily by children aged 0–19. Rate per thousand. Analysis by sex and age group, 1960–1973 (index 1964).

E.16 Mean duration of stay for children aged 0–19. Analysis by sex and age group, 1960–1973 (index 1964).

E.17 Duration of stay for children under 15. Analysis by age group showing percentage distribution of stay and estimated numbers, 1973 (index 1962).

E.18 Estimated numbers, percentages and discharge rates per 10,000 population aged under 15. Analysis by department and sex showing age group, 1973.

E.19 Discharge rates per 10,000 children under 15. Analysis by sex and Regional Hospital Board area of residence, 1960 and 1973 (index 1960).

6

E.20 Paediatric departments, average number of available beds. Analysis by Regional Health Authority area, 1975.

E.21 Infectious diseases departments, average number of available beds. Analysis by Regional Health Authority area, 1975.

E.22 Special care baby units. Analysis by Regional Health Authority area showing (a) number of beds and average duration of stay and (b) size of units, 1964 and 1971–1975.

E.23 Discharges from two regional centres with national comparisons. Analysis by diagnostic group, 1974.

E.24 Paediatric departments—day case and out-patient attendances. Analysis by Regional Hospital Board area, 1964 and 1972–1973 and by Regional Health Authority area, 1974 and 1975.

E.25 Casualty and out-patient departments. Attendances during a 3-month reference period, 1971–1973.

E.26 Accident and emergency departments and out-patient departments used by children. Analysis by extent of facilities for children and showing percentage having a qualified RSCN nurse, 1975.

E.27 Frenchay Hospital, Bristol: Accident and Emergency Department. Attendance by children aged 1–19 between March and September 1974. Analysis by primary diagnosis and age group.

E.28 Nottingham Children's Hospital: Accident and Emergency Department. Attendance by children under 15 in the year ending 31 March 1974. Analysis by nature of injury and age.

E.29 Mayday Hospital, Croydon: Accident and Emergency Department. Attendance by children under 19 in the year ending 31 December 1974. Analysis by diagnosis and age group.

E.30 Royal Hospital, Chesterfield: Out-Patient Department. Attendance by children under 15 in the year ending 31 December 1973. Analysis by diagnosis and age group.

Child Psychiatry

E.31 Resident patients aged under 15 and 15–19 in mental illness hospitals and units. Analysis by time spent in current hospital, 1954, 1963 and 1971.

E.32 Child psychiatry. Analysis by Regional Hospital Board area showing available beds, discharges and deaths, waiting list, new out-patients and total out-patient attendances, 1964 and 1971–1973 and by Regional Health Authority area, 1974.

E.33 Adolescent psychiatry. Analysis by Regional Hospital Board area showing available beds, discharges and deaths, waiting list, new out-patients and total out-patient attendances, 1972–1973 and by Regional Health Authority area, 1974.

E.34 Mental illness hospitals and units. Children and young people admitted. Analysis by age group showing numbers and rates, 1964 and 1970–1974.

E.35   Mental illness hospitals and units. Children and young people admitted for the first time. Analysis by age groups showing numbers and rates, 1964 and 1970–1974.

E.36   Mental handicap hospitals and units. Children under 15 admitted. Analysis by Regional Hospital Board area showing age group, sex, estimated numbers and rates, 1963 and 1973 and by Regional Health Authority area, 1974.

E.37   Mental handicap hospitals and units. Admissions. Analysis by sex and age group showing sex/age specific rates per 100,000 population, 1964 and 1970–1974.

F.   MANPOWER

General Medical and Dental Practitioners

F.1   General medical practitioners. Analysis by type of practitioner, 1965–1974.

F.2   Number of children aged 0–14 per general medical practitioner. Analysis by Regional Health Authority, 1974.

F.3   Number of unrestricted principals in group practice. Analysis by Standard Region, 1971–1974.

F.4   Number of health centres and number of places provided for general medical practitioners, 1966–1975.

F.5   General dental practitioners. Analysis by Regional Health Authority showing number and status of dentists and number of children aged 5–14 per dentist, 1974. National figures for 1964, 1969 and 1974.

Hospital Medical Staff

F.6   Hospital medical staff in paediatrics. Analysis by Regional Health Authority and grade showing number, wte and wte per 10,000 population at risk (i.e. children aged 0–14), 1974. National figures for 1964, 1969 and 1974.

F.7   Hospital medical staff in paediatric surgery. Analysis by Regional Health Authority and grade showing number, wte and wte per 10,000 live births, 1974. National figures for 1964, 1969 and 1974.

F.8   Hospital medical staff in mental illness—children. Analysis by Regional Health Authority and grade showing number, wte and wte per 10,000 population at risk (aged 0–19), 1974. National figures for 1964, 1969 and 1974.

Community Medical and Dental Staff

F.9   Medical staff in post with local health authorities—wte per 100,000 population aged 0–14, 1966–1973.

F.10   Medical and dental staff in the School Health Service, 1964–1974.

F.11   Community health medical staff. Analysis by grade and nature of contract, 1975.

Nurses

F.12 Community health nursing staff. Analysis by Regional Health Authority area and type of work showing number, wte and wte per 10,000 population, 1974.

F.13 Community health nursing staff. Analysis by type (health visitor, home nurse and midwife) showing case load for children under 5, 1963–1973.

F.14 Hospital nursing staff in post in wards containing children. Analysis by grade and nature of contract showing number and wte, 1975.

F.15 Hospital nursing staff in wards containing children. Analysis by grade, nature of contract and qualifications in children's nursing showing number and percentage qualified, 1975.

F.16 Student nurses in post in wards containing children. Analysis by grade of student nurse and course studied showing number and percentage of whole-time staff, 1975.

F.17 Number of medical schools, medical students and academic paediatric staff, 1970–1973. Great Britain.

G. REGIONAL AND AREA PROFILES

G.1 Child population, live birth rate (locally adjusted), child mortality rates, health service facilities (hospital beds, general practice and community nurses, including school nurses) by Regional and Area Health Authority.

Description of Regions (with maps)

The following symbols and abbreviations are used in the tables:

.. not available.

— nil or negligible.

. not applicable.

T Total.

M Male.

F Female.

Wte Whole-time equivalent.

ICD International statistical classification of diseases.

OPCS Office of Population Censuses and Surveys.

Section A

CHILD POPULATION

Tables A.1–6 provide some basic information on the number of children in England and Wales. For the purposes of this report the child population includes all under 16 and, additionally, those under 20 but still at school; for this reason, many of the tables relate to the age range 0–19. In any given year, the child population is a reflection of the pattern of births, deaths and migration for the previous 19 years. The Registrar General for England and Wales makes annual estimates of the population aged 0–19 by sex and single years of age and these estimates are given in Table A.1 for the years 1961, 1966, 1971, 1973 and 1974. The most reliable estimates are those made in the same year that a full population census is taken. Therefore, the figures for 1961 and 1971 represent the best estimates in this series. Such detailed annual estimates are not made below the national level but estimates for Regional Health Authority areas by sex and quinary age groups for 1973 and 1974 are available and are shown in Table A.3.

Population projections up to the year 1996 are shown in Table A.2. These are prepared by the Government Actuary in consultation with the Registrar General on the basis of an agreed set of assumptions about the future movements in fertility, mortality and external migration. The projections for England and Wales and Great Britain are most sensitive to the assumptions made on the future movement in the birth rate. Because of this a set of projections for Great Britain based on the mid-1974 population has been published using varying fertility assumptions, a selection of the statistics being shown in Table A.2, but it should be noted that there are no equivalent versions for England and Wales. Projecting numbers of live births presents many difficulties, particularly when there has been a recent change in direction in the trend. The downturn in births since 1964 led to a reduction in the expected number of live born children per woman incorporated in the projections.

In England and Wales in mid-1974, it was estimated that there were 15 million children under 20. This represents just over 30% of the total population. An estimated 11½ million were under 15 years of age.

The number and proportion of the population aged 0–19 increased steadily from 1951 but recently the effects of the fall in annual births since 1964 have reversed the trend; the child population of England and Wales is projected to fall to 14 million in 1986 (28% of total population) and although it is expected to reach nearly 15 million again by 1996, it may not exceed 12½ million if the continuing low variant projection for Great Britain applies for England and Wales. For the immediate future, the numbers aged 0–4, which have been falling since 1966, are projected to level off and subsequently rise in 1979, partly because the larger birth cohorts of 1950–1964 themselves enter the child bearing age groups and partly because fertility rates are projected to rise from the late 1970s. The same effect will influence, but somewhat later, the number of older children. Thus the 5–14s will reach a peak in 1976 and subsequently decline to 1986 while the 15–19 age group will not reach its peak till about 1981.

11

There are some regional variations in the proportion of total population falling in the age group 0–19. These are set out in Table A.3 for males and females separately for each new Regional Health Authority. The proportion is *lowest* in the four Thames Regions, East Anglian and South Western and *highest* in Mersey, Northern, Yorkshire, Wessex, Oxford and West Midlands.

Table A.4 shows the number of pupils in full- and part-time education and is of interest here in relation to the School Health Service. In 1974, there were 9·6 million full-time pupils aged from 2 to 15 and over, representing about 70% of the population aged 2–19. This table also sets out the proportion of children over school leaving age who are still at school and the extent to which the proportion has changed in the past 10 years. The school leaving age was raised to 16 in 1973 and this will have had some effect on the number of children remaining to later ages. Boys tend to stay on at school longer than girls but the gap has narrowed considerably in recent years. In 1974, some 27% of both boys and girls aged 16–17 were still at school but for the 18-year-olds about 8% of boys and 6% of girls had not left school.

About 30% of children live in the major conurbations of London, West Midlands, West Riding, Merseyside, South East Lancashire and Tyneside. Table A.5 shows that the proportion has declined slightly in the past 10 years, probably partly as a result of migration away from conurbations and partly as a result of the more rapid fall in the birthrate in conurbations, particularly London. These figures do not show, of course, the movement within conurbations as a result of redevelopment of the oldest parts.

An increasing proportion of the child population of England and Wales was born of parents who themselves were born outside the United Kingdom. Table A.6 shows that some 5% of all children aged 0–19 in 1971 were either born in the New Commonwealth or were born in the United Kingdom but had one or both parents born in the New Commonwealth[1]. Moreover, since birthplace of parents was first obtained at birth registration in 1969 the proportion of all births to parents of New Commonwealth or Pakistan origin has averaged about 6%. Table A.13 shows the most recent trends in the proportion of births by birthplace of mothers. Overall, between 1969 and 1974 about 11½% of all births were to women born outside the United Kingdom and a slightly increasing proportion born to mothers from the New Commonwealth and Pakistan (6·3% in 1974 compared with 5·9% in 1969). Table A.14 provides a regional analysis for 1974 and shows that births to New Commonwealth mothers are a much higher proportion of all births in the four Thames Regions and West Midlands than elsewhere.

Birth and Fertility Statistics

Table A.7 gives broad details of live birth rates by legitimacy for each year since 1951. Live births per 1,000 women aged 15–44 rose steadily from 73 in 1955 to a peak of 93 in 1964 since when there has been a steady decline particularly marked in the last few years so that the 1975 figure stood at 63·3—the lowest peacetime level reached since the mid-30s, when the rate fell to 59 in 1933.

---

[1]"New Commonwealth" as defined in 1971, ie including Pakistan.

This decline in fertility has been observed in all regions and Table A.8 sets out details of the changes between 1963 and 1973 for Hospital Regions[1]. There is a marked variation in the absolute rates and also in the extent to which these have declined. One noticeable fact is that total period fertility rates were lowest in 1973 in the four metropolitan regions and in two of these, the NW and SW Metropolitan Regions, greater than average declines in fertility rates over the previous 10 years occurred. The converse is noticeable in Wales, West Midlands, Leeds and East Anglian.

The number of illegitimate births reached a peak in 1967–68 at about 70,000 and has subsequently declined although accounting for a higher proportion of all births in 1974 (8·8%) than in 1964 (7·2%). The number of children born within the first eight months of marriage, and defined in the statistics to be pre-maritally conceived, were some 12,000 lower in 1973 than in 1963 but accounted for much the same proportion of births (8%) at the two dates. Overall, therefore, there has been a decline in the number of births conceived outside marriage but these now represent a slightly higher proportion of all births—16·3% in 1973 compared to 14·5% in 1963. Table A.9 sets out the considerable increases in the proportion of illegitimate births in the Newcastle, Welsh, Manchester and Liverpool Hospital Regions between 1963 and 1973; in two of these, Newcastle and Liverpool, the proportion of pre-maritally conceived births also rose. By contrast in East Anglian, three of the Metropolitan Regions and in the Oxford Region the overall proportion of extra-maritally conceived babies declined. The explanation of these variations is complex but may partly lie in the fact that attitudes towards abortion are more favourable in some regions than others. Abortion seems to be least popular in regions where the proportion of extra-maritally conceived births has shown most increase. Another factor influencing the number of illegitimate births compared with pre-maritally conceived births is the proportion of single girls who become pregnant and marry before the baby is born. Again, regional differences in attitude to marriage in these circumstances may explain much of the variation. Whatever the reason for these variations, unmarried mothers and their children are known to present additional problems to health services.

Table A.10 illustrates the continuing trend in recent years for confinements to take place in hospital. In 1966, 72·2% of all live and still births were in NHS hospitals and by 1973 the percentage had reached 92·1. The fall in the birth rate has clearly facilitated this trend.

Table A.11 examines, at national level, the changes in the birth rate between 1964, 1971, 1973 and 1974 by age of mother. The decline in fertility during this period has been characterised by a particularly marked decline in the rates for older women and a concentration of childbearing within the age group 20–29. Rates for women aged 30–34 have almost halved while those for women 40–44 have more than halved, accounting in 1973 for only 1·4% of live births. In contrast, the rates for 15–19 year olds show some small increase. Another characteristic of the decline in fertility is set out in Table A.12 which shows the number and proportion of high parity births, defined as fifth or later children,

---

[1]ie the hospital region in which the mother lived.

have also considerably declined. Better family planning facilities and the availability of legal abortion must have played a part in this decline and certainly reduced the number of births to women over 40 years of age.

The way in which these annual changes have affected the pattern of childbearing in different marriage groups can be illustrated by the following summary tables. Table A shows how there has been a marked change since the mid-1960s in the proportion of women who have not had a child after two years of their first marriage—this increase is observed for brides of all ages but most markedly for those aged 20–24. Table B shows the decline in the proportion of large families.

Table A

PERCENTAGE OF FIRST MARRIAGES WITH NO CHILD AFTER TWO YEARS—BY AGE OF WIFE AND YEAR OF MARRIAGE: ENGLAND AND WALES

	Year of Marriage				
	1951	1956	1961	1966	1971
All marriages under 45	49·7	46·3	42·5	45·0	56·3
under 20	33·7	32·4	28·5	31·6	40·6
20–24	51·8	50·0	47·7	52·0	65·1
25–29	51.9	48·5	45·2	48·5	58·8
30–34	53·0	48·2	45·9	49·1	53·2
35–39	66·7	61·7	58·8	61·2	63·9

Source: OPCS

Table B

PROPORTION (PER THOUSAND) OF WOMEN, MARRIED ONCE ONLY AT AGES 20–24, WITH THREE OR MORE CHILDREN AFTER 10 YEARS OF MARRIAGE: ENGLAND AND WALES

	Year of Marriage				
	1951	1956	1961	1963	1964
Number of Children	Proportion (per thousand)				
3	155	189	215	206	190
4	53	71	63	59	50
5 or more	30	36	25	19	15

Source: OPCS

Tables A.15 and 16 give data on births and abortions to the under-20s which are of particular concern to the committee. The relationships between contraception, abortion and birth, within and outside marriage, is complex, particularly for this age group. However, the general picture of the trend in births

14

and abortions suggests that this group have been affected less by the growth in family planning than other groups. Nothing is known, of course, about the prevalence of illegal abortion before or after the 1967 Abortion Act although it is generally believed that the increase in legal abortions—up to 1970 at least—contained a large element of transfer from the "illegal" sector.

Although since 1971 the decline in the illegitimate birth rate was more than compensated by increases in legal abortions for girls under 20, the most recent evidence suggests that, when all extra-marital pregnancies are considered and allowance is made for the interval between the foetal age at which an abortion is normally carried out and the full gestational length of a normal confinement, the " total pregnancy rate " for girls under 20 reached a peak in 1972 and has fallen since then. The fall is most marked among older girls and the conclusion is that contraceptive advice is now being taken and acted upon. There is little evidence of a similar fall for girls of 17 and younger as yet.

ESTIMATED HOME POPULATION¹ IN SINGLE YEARS AND AGE GROUPS 0–19—1961, 1966, 1971, 1973 and 1974

Age Group 0–19 as Percentage of Home Population

Table A.1

England and Wales

Thousands

Age (in years)	As at 30 June 1961			As at 30 June 1966			As at 30 June 1971			As at 30 June 1973			As at 30 June 1974		
	Persons	Males	Females	Persons	Males	Females	Persons	Males	Females	Persons	Males	Females	Persons	Males	Females
All ages	46,196	22,347	23,849	47,824	23,209	24,615	48,854	23,737	25,117	49,175	23,916	25,259	49,201	23,940	25,261
0–19	13,856	7,084	6,772	14,736	7,541	7,195	14,926	7,658	7,268	15,026	7,708	7,317	14,973	7,680	7,293
Percentage of home population	30·0	31·7	28·4	30·8	32·5	29·2	30·6	32·3	28·9	30·6	32·2	29·0	30·4	32·1	29·9
0	783	402	380	835	427	409	779	400	379	690	355	335	641	329	311
1	744	383	362	846	433	413	758	389	369	735	379	356	687	354	334
2	729	374	355	840	430	410	782	401	382	774	396	378	733	378	355
3	713	366	347	822	420	403	780	400	380	752	386	366	772	395	377
4	686	352	334	806	413	394	807	414	392	781	400	381	750	386	365
0–4	3,656	1,878	1,778	4,150	2,122	2,028	3,905	2,004	1,902	3,733	1,917	1,816	3,583	1,841	1,741
5	662	340	322	777	399	378	810	415	395	775	398	377	773	399	380
6	647	332	315	741	381	360	826	424	402	805	413	393	773	396	376
7	657	337	321	728	374	353	824	422	401	807	414	394	804	412	392
8	650	333	317	712	366	346	805	413	392	825	423	402	806	413	393
9	648	332	316	687	355	332	789	405	384	823	422	401	823	422	401
5–9	3,264	1,672	1,592	3,645	1,876	1,769	4,053	2,079	1,974	4,036	2,069	1,967	3,984	2,042	1,942
10	662	339	323	663	343	320	768	395	373	804	412	392	823	423	401
11	688	352	336	648	333	314	738	380	359	790	405	385	804	412	392
12	719	368	350	661	341	320	729	374	354	771	396	375	790	405	384
13	783	400	383	652	335	317	715	367	347	740	380	359	770	396	374
14	834	426	407	646	329	317	695	358	337	729	374	354	739	380	359
10–14	3,686	1,887	1,799	3,270	1,682	1,588	3,645	1,874	1,771	3,834	1,968	1,866	3,926	2,016	1,910
15	683	349	334	663	338	326	674	347	326	718	369	349	719	375	356
16	675	344	330	687	350	337	654	337	317	696	356	339	719	369	350
17	667	339	328	717	366	352	674	346	327	674	344	329	697	356	341
18	642	324	319	768	388	381	666	340	327	657	337	321	675	344	330
19	583	291	292	835	420	415	654	331	323	679	348	331	659	337	321
15–19	3,250	1,647	1,603	3,671	1,861	1,810	3,322	1,702	1,621	3,423	1,754	1,669	3,480	1,781	1,700

¹Population of all types actually in England and Wales, revised in the light of the results of the 1971 Census.
All figures have been independently rounded.

Source: OPCS

PROJECTED TOTAL POPULATION BY AGE 1974–1996; MID-1974 BASED PROJECTIONS

Table A.2   Thousands

Age-group	1976	1981	1986	1991	1996
GREAT BRITAIN					
a. High variant; with migration					
All ages	54,605	55,356	56,397	57,618	58,750
0–19	16,617	16,616	16,572	16,963	17,922
0– 4	3,681	4,135	4,525	4,743	4,646
5– 9	4,307	3,641	4,092	4,481	4,698
10–14	4,512	4,298	3,630	4,081	4,470
15–19	4,117	4,542	4,325	3,658	4,108
b. Central projection; with migration					
All ages	54,542	54,700	55,537	56,572	57,499
0–19	16,555	15,961	15,712	15,916	16,732
0– 4	3,619	3,542	4,318	4,554	4,439
5– 9	4,307	3,579	3,500	4,275	4,511
10–14	4,512	4,298	3,569	3,490	4,264
15–19	4,117	4,542	4,325	3,597	3,518
c. Low variant; with migration					
All ages	54,512	54,263	54,842	55,652	56,348
0–19	16,525	15,523	15,018	14,995	15,611
0– 4	3,589	3,134	4,059	4,328	4,207
5– 9	4,307	3,549	3,094	4,016	4,285
10–14	4,512	4,298	3,540	3,084	4,006
15–19	4,117	4,542	4,325	3,567	3,113
d. Continuing low variant; with migration					
All ages	54,512	54,251	54,308	54, 497	54,590
0–19	16,525	15,512	14,483	13,842	13,852
0– 4	3,589	3,123	3,536	3,707	3,602
5– 9	4,307	3,549	3,082	3,495	3,665
10–14	4,512	4,298	3,540	3,073	3,484
15–19	4,117	4,542	4,325	3,567	3,101
ENGLAND AND WALES					
b. Central projection; with migration					
All ages	49,282	49,387	50,077	50,941	51,713
0–19	14,853	14,336	14,091	14,242	14,942
0– 4	3,259	3,169	3,848	4,059	3,962
5– 9	3,871	3,226	3,134	3,812	4,022
10–14	4,048	3,866	3,219	3,127	3,805
15–19	3,675	4,075	3,890	3,244	3,153
0–19 as % of home population	30·1	29·0	28·1	28·0	28·9

Source: OPCS

Variant population projections 1974–2011 prepared by the Government Actuary.

ESTIMATED HOME POPULATION UNDER 20 YEARS OF AGE

By Regional Health Authority, Sex and Age Groups—30 June 1973 and 1974

Percentages of Regional Population of all Ages of the same Sex.

Table A.3

England and Wales

MALES

Regional Health Authority	30 June 1973							30 June 1974						
	Numbers (thousands)	Percentages						Numbers (thousands)	Percentages					
	All ages	<1	1–4	5–9	10–14	15–19	0–19	All ages	<1	1–4	5–9	10–14	15–19	0–19
England and Wales ...	23,915·8	1·5	6·5	8·7	8·2	7·3	32·2	23,940·3	1·4	6·3	8·5	8·4	7·4	32·1
Northern	1,528·4	1·4	6·5	8·8	8·8	7·8	33·4	1,526·8	1·3	6·2	8·7	9·0	7·8	33·0
Yorkshire	1,733·7	1·5	6·7	8·7	8·4	7·6	32·9	1,737·8	1·4	6·5	8·7	8·5	7·7	32·8
Trent	2,232·4	1·5	6·7	8·7	8·2	7·3	32·4	2,236·8	1·4	6·5	8·6	8·4	7·4	32·3
East Anglian ...	861·0	1·5	6·4	8·4	7·9	7·1	31·3	869·5	1·4	6·3	8·3	8·0	7·1	31·2
NW Thames ...	1,713·7	1·4	6·0	8·0	7·6	6·9	30·0	1,696·5	1·3	5·8	7·9	7·9	7·0	30·0
NE Thames ...	1,820·5	1·5	6·4	8·4	7·8	7·0	31·1	1,810·6	1·4	6·2	8·3	8·0	7·1	30·9
SE Thames ...	1,731·4	1·4	6·3	8·5	8·0	7·2	31·4	1,726·7	1·3	6·1	8·4	8·2	7·1	31·1
SW Thames ...	1,384·8	1·3	5·9	8·2	7·9	7·2	30·5	1,380·6	1·2	5·7	8·0	8·1	7·3	30·3
Wessex	1,263·8	1·5	6·7	8·9	8·4	7·3	32·8	1,276·8	1·4	6·5	8·7	8·5	7·9	33·0
Oxford	1,071·5	1·6	6·9	9·3	8·5	7·6	33·9	1,086·0	1·5	6·7	9·2	8·7	7·8	33·7
South Western ...	1,496·6	1·4	6·1	8·3	8·0	7·3	31·1	1,506·2	1·4	5·9	8·2	8·1	7·4	31·0
West Midlands ...	2,556·1	1·5	7·0	9·0	8·4	7·5	33·3	2,564·6	1·4	6·7	8·9	8·6	7·5	33·1
Mersey	1,215·7	1·5	7·0	9·3	9·3	7·8	34·9	1,214·0	1·4	6·7	9·2	9·4	7·9	34·5
North Western ...	1,972·7	1·5	6·8	8·8	8·2	7·1	32·5	1,969·7	1·4	6·6	8·7	8·5	7·3	32·5
Wales	1,333·5	1·5	6·5	8·6	8·3	7·4	32·2	1,337·7	1·4	6·3	8·4	8·5	7·5	32·1

FEMALES

	25,258·8	1·3	5·9	7·8	7·4	6·6	29·0	25,260·9	1·2	5·7	7·7	7·6	6·7	28·9
England and Wales ...														
Northern ...	1,603·9	1·3	5·8	8·0	8·0	7·1	30·4	1,601·9	1·2	5·6	7·9	8·2	7·2	30·1
Yorkshire ...	1,837·9	1·4	6·1	7·9	7·5	6·6	29·4	1,841·5	1·2	5·9	7·8	7·7	6·7	29·3
Trent ...	2,294·9	1·4	6·2	8·1	7·6	6·7	30·0	2,299·9	1·3	6·0	8·0	7·8	6·8	29·9
East Anglian ...	878·0	1·4	5·9	7·8	7·1	6·5	28·7	888·7	1·4	5·8	7·7	7·3	6·5	28·7
NW Thames ...	1,804·5	1·3	5·4	7·2	6·9	6·4	27·1	1,789·2	1·2	5·3	7·1	7·1	6·6	27·2
NE Thames ...	1,935·5	1·3	5·7	7·5	6·9	6·5	27·9	1,923·6	1·2	5·5	7·4	7·1	6·6	27·9
SE Thames ...	1,905·4	1·2	5·4	7·3	6·9	6·3	27·1	1,896·2	1·1	5·2	7·2	7·1	6·4	27·0
SW Thames ...	1,520·1	1·2	5·1	7·1	6·8	6·3	26·5	1,510·9	1·1	5·0	6·9	7·0	6·4	26·4
Wessex ...	1,335·6	1·4	6·0	7·9	7·5	6·5	29·2	1,345·5	1·2	5·7	7·8	7·6	6·6	29·1
Oxford ...	1,087·2	1·5	6·4	8·6	7·9	6·8	31·2	1,097·5	1·4	6·3	8·4	8·1	7·0	31·1
South Western ...	1,612·1	1·2	5·4	7·3	7·0	6·4	27·3	1,622·5	1·2	5·2	7·2	7·1	6·5	27·2
West Midlands ...	2,607·1	1·4	6·5	8·4	7·7	6·8	30·8	2,614·8	1·3	6·2	8·3	7·9	6·9	30·6
Mersey ...	1,300·8	1·4	6·1	8·3	8·3	7·1	31·2	1,296·3	1·2	5·9	8·2	8·4	7·3	30·9
North Western ...	2,120·0	1·3	6·0	7·8	7·4	6·3	28·8	2,112·9	1·2	5·7	7·7	7·6	6·5	28·8
Wales ...	1,415·8	1·3	5·8	7·7	7·5	6·8	29·1	1,419·5	1·2	5·6	7·6	7·6	6·9	29·0

Source: OPCS/DHSS.

19

CHILDREN AT SCHOOL

Numbers: Percentage remaining at school beyond the statutory leaving age—At January in 1964–1974

Table A.4

NUMBERS

	1964	1965	1966	1967	1968	1969	1970	1971	1972	1973	1974
Full-time pupils											
In all schools											
Total	7,711,529	7,759,816	7,844,648	7,980,940	8,183,237	8,391,756	8,597,451	8,800,843	9,032,999	9,190,030	9,560,015
Aged 2–4	222,407	237,053	237,907	237,502	247,101	256,231	263,771	278,545	299,200	327,987	337,536
Aged 5–14	6,708,137	6,737,742	6,824,714	6,953,060	7,112,722	7,277,265	7,457,993	7,632,691	7,800,860	7,897,613	7,958,502
Aged 15 and over	780,985	785,021	782,027	790,378	823,414	858,260	875,687	889,607	932,939	964,430	1,263,977
In maintained schools (other than nursery and special)											
Total	7,033,696	7,092,155	7,183,165	7,328,110	7,541,969	7,753,002	7,960,194	8,167,009	8,366,333	8,513,728	8,872,567
Aged 15 and over	635,307	641,106	641,279	653,105	687,131	721,912	740,647	755,439	793,171	821,399	1,115,603
In maintained nursery schools	20,580	19,926	19,417	19,039	17,957	17,170	16,441	15,596	15,443	15,450	15,431
In all special schools											
Total	72,541	74,299	76,466	78,256	81,678	84,812	86,847	90,361	122,283	127,804	130,677
Aged 15 and over	9,287	9,389	9,725	9,729	10,314	10,751	10,595	10,945	15,922	17,517	19,761
In direct grant schools (other than special)											
Total	115,369	116,123	116,776	118,027	119,346	119,523	120,181	119,483	119,865	121,384	122,193
Aged 15 and over	41,371	42,160	41,792	42,420	43,259	43,598	44,032	43,975	44,671	45,415	46,041
In independent schools recognised as efficient											
Total	307,624	306,587	308,834	305,421	299,883	301,166	303,977	305,533	311,116	315,391	324,326
Aged 15 and over	77,596	77,037	76,621	74,282	73,363	73,287	72,978	72,961	73,295	64,103	76,055
In other independent schools											
Total	161,719	150,726	139,990	132,087	122,404	116,083	109,811	102,861	97,959	96,273	94,821
Aged 15 and over	17,424	15,329	12,610	10,842	9,347	8,712	7,435	6,287	5,880	5,996	6,517

In all schools ...	25,020	29,991	32,761	37,096	44,411	53,468	60,707	72,392	86,441	101,065	122,326
In maintained primary schools ...	7,421	10,431	11,382	13,876	16,857	22,778	28,520	37,547	48,257	59,660	77,972
In maintained nursery schools ...	6,184	7,975	9,044	10,385	12,716	15,070	17,779	20,718	23,998	26,947	30,401
In all special schools ...	··	··	··	··	··	··	48	70	341	315	354
In direct grant schools ...	581	420	434	484	535	610	664	620	611	418	398
In independent schools recognised as efficient ...	2,236	2,504	2,743	2,703	3,634	3,957	3,797	3,854	4,076	4,396	4,400
In other independent schools ...	8,598	8,661	9,158	9,648	10,669	11,053	9,899	9,583	9,158	9,329	8,801

PERCENTAGE REMAINING AT SCHOOL BEYOND THE STATUTORY LEAVING AGE[1]

Boys and Girls											
15 ...	41·2	44·3	47·1	50·2	53·6	56·2	57·7	59·1	60·6	61·3	·
16 ...	24·9	26·8	28·6	30·3	32·6	34·5	35·5	36·2	37·5	37·2	26·8
17 ...	13·5	13·9	15·1	16·5	17·9	19·1	20·1	20·6	21·2	21·6	20·8
18 ...	4·4	4·9	4·9	5·5	6·0	6·3	6·5	6·8	6·9	6·9	6·9
19 and over ...	0·4	0·4	0·5	0·5	0·6	0·6	0·6	0·6	0·6	0·6	0·5
Boys											
15 ...	41·8	44·6	47·4	50·7	54·1	56·7	58·1	59·6	61·2	61·5	·
16 ...	26·5	28·3	29·8	31·4	33·6	35·3	36·3	36·9	38·2	37·7	26·8
17 ...	15·2	15·6	16·7	17·9	19·1	20·2	21·0	21·4	21·9	22·3	21·2
18 ...	5·7	6·1	6·1	6·7	7·2	7·4	7·6	7·8	8·0	7·8	7·7
19 and over ...	0·7	0·7	0·7	0·8	0·9	0·9	0·8	0·8	0·9	0·8	0·7
Girls											
15 ...	40·6	43·9	46·7	49·7	53·0	55·7	57·3	58·5	59·9	61·0	·
16 ...	23·3	25·3	27·3	29·2	31·6	33·6	34·6	35·5	36·8	36·7	26·8
17 ...	11·8	12·2	13·5	15·0	16·5	17·9	19·2	19·7	20·5	21·0	20·4
18 ...	3·1	3·6	3·6	4·1	4·7	5·1	5·3	5·7	5·8	6·0	6·0
19 and over ...	0·2	0·2	0·2	0·2	0·3	0·3	0·3	0·3	0·3	0·3	0·3

Source: Department of Education and Science

[1] All schools excluding special schools. In January of year shown; age at the beginning of January. The number of pupils aged 15, 16, 17, 18 and over expressed as a percentage of the 13-year-old pupils 2, 3, 4 and 5 years earlier respectively. Since January 1964, 15-year-olds in England and Wales have been over school-leaving age only if born between January and August, as in 1963 the Christmas leaving date was abolished. For the 15-year-old age group, therefore, the figures for England and Wales for 1964 and later years are restricted to those born between January and August.

The raising of the school-leaving age affected the 16-year-old age group and led to a break in the continuity of the series for that age group between 1973 and 1974.

ESTIMATED HOME POPULATION BY URBAN/RURAL AGGREGATES—30 JUNE 1963 AND 1973

Table A.5

England and Wales
Thousands

MALES

Population living in	No./%	30 June 1963 All ages	Total 0–19	Under 1	1–4	5–9	10–14	15–19	30 June 1973 All ages	Total 0–19	Under 1	1–4	5–9	10–14	15–19
1. Conurbations	No.	8,104·1	2,523·5	157·2	559·7	595·1	595·0	616·5	7,623·7	2,393·1	112·2	483·5	635·8	607·6	554·0
	%	35·5	34·4	37·0	35·5	34·3	34·3	33·1	31·9	31·0	31·6	31·0	30·7	30·9	31·6
Areas outside Conurbations:															
2. Urban areas with populations of 100,000 or more	No.	3,039·4	984·7	56·8	215·1	234·7	235·1	243·0	3,136·1	1,007·0	46·5	197·9	265·8	257·8	239·0
	%	13·3	13·4	13·4	13·6	13·5	13·5	13·0	13·1	13·1	13·1	12·7	12·8	13·1	13·6
3. Urban areas with populations of 50,000 and under 100,000	No.	2,101·7	679·5	38·4	146·5	160·5	161·1	173·0	2,355·6	771·9	34·6	153·5	206·3	199·9	177·6
	%	9·2	9·3	9·0	9·3	9·2	9·3	9·3	9·8	10·0	9·7	9·8	10·0	10·2	10·1
4. Urban areas with populations of less than 50,000	No.	4,718·1	1,525·5	86·7	331·4	370·0	370·1	367·3	5,360·1	1,752·9	80·9	361·2	476·1	445·2	389·5
	%	20·7	20·8	20·4	21·0	21·3	21·3	19·7	22·4	22·7	22·8	23·1	23·0	22·6	22·2
5. Rural Districts	No.	4,868·2	1,624·6	85·4	324·2	376·3	375·9	462·8	5,440·3	1,783·6	81·1	365·6	485·4	457·4	394·1
	%	21·3	22·1	20·1	20·6	21·7	21·6	24·8	22·7	23·1	22·8	23·4	23·5	23·2	22·5
6. All Areas	No.	22,831·5	7,337·8	424·5	1,576·9	1,736·6	1,737·2	1,862·6	23,915·8	7,708·5	355·3	1,561·7	2,069·4	1,967·9	1,754·2
	%	100·0	100·0	100·0	100·0	100·0	100·0	100·0	100·0	100·0	100·0	100·0	100·0	100·0	100·0

FEMALES

Population living in	No./%	30 June 1963 All ages	Total 0–19	Under 1	1–4	5–9	10–14	15–19	30 June 1973 All ages	Total 0–19	Under 1	1–4	5–9	10–14	15–19
1. Conurbations	No.	8,878·7	2,467·3	149·1	530·8	571·0	571·6	644·8	8,155·7	2,293·8	105·8	458·8	610·1	581·4	537·7
	%	36·7	35·3	37·0	35·5	34·7	34·7	36·0	32·3	31·3	31·6	31·0	31·0	31·2	32·2
Areas outside Conurbations:															
2. Urban areas with populations of 100,000 or more	No.	3,253·2	957·8	54·2	205·5	225·4	225·5	247·2	3,324·5	962·5	43·7	189·8	254·7	246·6	227·7
	%	13·4	13·7	13·5	13·7	13·7	13·7	13·8	13·2	13·2	13·0	12·8	13·0	13·2	13·6
3. Urban areas with populations of 50,000 and less than 100,000	No.	2,271·8	647·1	36·1	138·0	153·0	153·5	166·5	2,525·7	734·7	33·0	144·8	196·5	190·7	169·7
	%	9·4	9·3	9·0	9·2	9·3	9·3	9·3	10·0	10·0	9·8	9·8	10·0	10·2	10·2
4. Urban areas with populations of less than 50,000	No.	5,030·9	1,469·8	82·5	314·0	348·8	349·2	375·3	5,728·8	1,668·5	76·4	342·2	450·7	424·1	375·1
	%	20·8	21·0	20·5	21·0	21·2	21·2	21·0	22·7	22·8	22·8	23·1	22·9	22·7	22·5
5. Rural Districts	No.	4,756·6	1,441·8	80·9	306·6	348·5	349·4	356·4	5,524·1	1,657·8	76·2	345·4	454·7	423·0	358·5
	%	19·7	20·6	20·1	20·5	21·2	21·2	19·9	21·9	22·7	22·7	23·3	23·1	22·1	21·5
6. All Areas	No.	24,191·2	6,983·8	402·8	1,494·9	1,646·7	1,649·2	1,790·2	25,258·8	7,317·3	335·1	1,481·0	1,966·7	1,865·8	1,668·7
	%	100·0	100·0	100·0	100·0	100·0	100·0	100·0	100·0	100·0	100·0	100·0	100·0	100·0	100·0

Source: OPCS

NOTE: These aggregates comprise (1) the conurbations of Greater London, Tyneside, West Midlands, West Yorkshire, South-East Lancashire and Merseyside as defined by the Registrar General (2) the aggregates of urban local authorities outside the conurbations in three groups according to their resident population in April 1961 and (3) the aggregate of rural local authority areas outside conurbations. Urban areas include Boroughs and Urban Districts as defined by the Local Government Acts prior to 1 April 1974 and rural areas are rural districts similarly defined. The estimates for mid-1963 and mid-1973 are based on the results of the 1961 and 1971 censuses respectively.

Table A.6   **England and Wales**

Country of Birth of E	10–14 Females		15–19 Males		Females	
	No.	%	No.	%	No.	%
ALL COUNTRIES OF BIR)	1,759,550	100·0	1,689,585	100·0	1,610,215	100·0
A. INDIVIDUAL BORN (BOTH PARENTS B(ISLES[2]						
TOTAL ...;	55,985	3·2	87,320	5·2	74,760	4·6
Individual Born:						
Irish Republi	5,280	0·3	10,895	0·6	11,780	0·7
Old Common	1,825	0·1	1,480	0·1	1,830	0·1
New Commo	36,140	2·1	59,485	3·5	43,480	2·7
India ...;	7,360	0·4	14,185	0·8	10,390	0·6
Pakistan;	3,415	0·2	15,460	0·9	2,905	0·2
African (	8,090	0·5	9,150	0·5	7,765	0·5
Americai	12,190	0·7	13,515	0·8	15,540	1·0
Mediterr;	2,825	0·2	3,660	0·2	3,530	0·2
Remaind	2,260	0·1	3,515	0·2	3,350	0·2
Other Foreig	12,740	0·7	15,460	0·9	17,670	1·1
B. INDIVIDUAL BORN BORN OUTSIDE U						
TOTAL ...;	62,325	3·5	35,335	2·1	34,330	2·1
Both Parents Bor						
Irish Republi	25,370	1·4	17,500	1·0	16,770	1·0
Old Common	155	0·0	105	0·0	135	0·0
New Commo	19,995	1·1	3,950	0·2	3,760	0·2
India ...	2,590	0·1	1,060	0·1	965	0·1
Pakistan)	260	0·0	95	0·0	60	0·0
African (	295	0·0	100	0·0	90	0·0
Americar	13,715	0·8	1,135	0·1	1,215	0·1
Mediterr;	2,620	0·1	1,320	0·1	1,235	0·1
Remaind)	115	0·0	45	0·0	45	0·0
Different)	395	0·0	200	0·0	150	0·0
One Parent b(elsewhere[6]	2,695	0·2	1,595	0·1	1,510	0·1
Other Combi	14,110	0·8	12,190	0·7	12,150	0·8
C. INDIVIDUAL BORN BORN UK, OTI OUTSIDE UK						
TOTAL ...;	110,885	6·3	103,135	6·1	99,220	6·2
One Parent born (						
Irish Republi	43,615	2·5	38,015	2·2	36,910	2·3
Old Common	6,045	0·3	6,960	0·4	6,755	0·4
New Commo	18,720	1·1	13,300	0·8	12,835	0·8
India ...	7,670	0·4	6,305	0·4	6,090	0·4
Pakistan	1,275	0·1	1,025	0·1	985	0·1
African (	1,550	0·1	1,070	0·1	1,025	0·1
Americar	3,400	0·2	1,550	0·1	1,525	0·1
Mediterr;	3,095	0·2	2,110	0·1	2,035	0·1
Remaind(	1,725	0·1	1,245	0·1	1,175	0·1
Other Foreign	42,505	2·4	44,860	2·7	42,720	2·7

1. Total enumerated ;
2. Includes all person;
3. Includes Pakistan.
4. Includes Rhodesia.
5. Irish Republic, Ol(
6. Both Foreign; one

Source: OPCS
Census 1971

There is an additional is amounts to some 500,000 children or 3·4 per cent of all children.
0–19. A certain prop(heir parents) but of New Commonwealth "origin" as a proportion of all
children with a stated ;
Figures may not add t(

24

LIVE BIRTH RATES BY LEGITIMACY—1951 to 1975

Table A.7

England and Wales

Year	Number of live births (thousands)			Total live births per 1,000 population of all ages	Total live births per 1,000 women aged 15–44	Legitimate births per 1,000 married women aged 15–44	Illegitimate births per 1,000 unmarried women aged 15–44	Illegitimate births per 1,000 total live births	Male births per 1,000 female births		
	Persons	Males	Females						Total births	Legitimate births	Illegitimate births
1951	677·5	348·6	328·9	15·5	71·6	105·5	9·8	48	1,060	1,060	1,060
1952	673·7	345·9	327·9	15·3	71·8	104·6	10·0	48	1,055	1,054	1,066
1953	684·4	352·0	332·3	15·5	73·5	106·4	10·2	47	1,059	1,059	1,062
1954	673·7	346·5	327·2	15·2	72·9	104·8	10·2	47	1,059	1,059	1,059
1955	667·8	343·7	324·1	15·0	72·8	103·7	10·3	47	1,060	1,060	1,058
1956	700·3	359·9	340·5	15·7	77·0	108·2	11·4	48	1,057	1,057	1,055
1957	723·4	372·3	351·1	16·1	80·0	111·7	12·0	48	1,060	1,061	1,049
1958	740·7	380·9	359·8	16·4	82·1	114·3	12·7	49	1,059	1,059	1,055
1959	748·5	385·7	362·8	16·5	83·0	115·4	13·3	51	1,063	1,063	1,069
1960	785·0	404·2	380·9	17·1	86·8	120·8	14·7	54	1,061	1,062	1,048
1961	811·3	417·8	393·5	17·6	89·2	123·8	16·5	60	1,062	1,062	1,063
1962	838·7	431·6	407·1	18·0	90·7	126·1	18·3	66	1,060	1,060	1,058
1963	854·1	438·5	415·6	18·2	91·3	126·9	19·1	69	1,055	1,056	1,046
1964	876·0	451·1	424·9	18·6	93·0	128·7	20·4	72	1,062	1,061	1,069
1965	862·7	443·2	419·5	18·1	92·1	126·9	21·4	77	1,056	1,056	1,059
1966	849·8	437·3	412·6	17·8	90·8	124·8	21·7	79	1,060	1,061	1,053
1967	832·2	427·9	404·3	17·3	89·1	121·5	22·8	84	1,058	1,059	1,048
1968	819·3	421·1	398·1	16·9	87·9	119·2	23·0	85	1,058	1,058	1,054
1969	797·5	410·1	387·5	16·4	85·6	115·8	22·3	84	1,058	1,059	1,054
1970	784·5	403·4	381·1	16·1	84·3	113·5	21·8	83	1,058	1,058	1,058
1971	783·2	403·2	379·9	16·0	84·0	112·4	22·3	84	1,061	1,060	1,072
1972	725·4	374·0	351·5	14·8	77·5	103·6	21·1	86	1,064	1,064	1,070
1973	676·0	348·7	327·3	13·7	71·7	96·2	19·3	86	1,065	1,065	1,067
1974	639·9	329·5	310·4	13·0	67·5	91·1	18·4	88	1,061	1,060	1,070
1975	603·4	310·8	292·7	12·3	63·3	85·8	17·5	91	1,062	1,062	1,061

25

BIRTH RATES AND FERTILITY RATES 1963–1974

Table A.8

a. by Hospital Region—1963, 1971 and 1973

England and Wales

Hospital Region	Total live births (thousands) 1973	Birth rate per 1,000 home population of all ages				Total period fertility rates				Illegitimate births (thousands) 1973	Extra-maritally conceived births[1] (thousands) 1973
		1963	1971	1973	Index (1963=100) 1973	1963	1971	1973	Index (1963=100) 1973	1973	1973
England and Wales ...	676·0	18·2	16·0	13·7	75	2·85	2·40	2·03	71	58·1	110·4
Newcastle	41·1	18·5	16·1	13·5	73	2·88	2·48	2·04	71	3·7	7·8
Leeds	44·9	17·9	16·4	13·8	77	2·85	2·54	2·12	74	4·4	8·3
Sheffield	65·9	18·5	16·7	14·0	76	2·91	2·50	2·08	71	5·7	11·2
East Anglian ...	26·5	17·0	15·9	14·5	85	2·71	2·36	2·14	79	1·7	3·4
NW Metropolitan ...	56·3	18·9	15·5	13·3	70	2·91	2·12	1·80	62	5·2	8·7
NE Metropolitan ...	46·3	18·1	16·2	14·1	78	2·79	2·37	2·05	73	3·6	6·3
SE Metropolitan ...	44·1	17·3	14·7	12·8	74	2·65	2·27	1·96	74	3·6	6·4
SW Metropolitan ...	41·4	17·1	14·6	12·6	74	2·63	2·08	1·77	67	4·2	6·9
Wessex	28·0	17·7	15·3	13·3	75	2·94	2·33	2·01	68	2·1	3·9
Oxford	31·1	19·7	17·2	15·1	77	3·28	2·44	2·08	63	1·9	3·7
South Western ...	42·8	17·0	15·0	13·2	78	2·87	2·35	2·07	72	3·3	6·5
Birmingham	74·9	19·0	17·2	14·5	76	2·83	2·55	2·12	75	6·0	11·6
Manchester	63·3	18·0	16·4	13·8	77	2·95	2·54	2·10	71	6·6	12·4
Liverpool	31·1	20·0	16·9	14·1	70	3·02	2·58	2·12	70	3·0	6·3
Welsh	37·6	17·7	15·8	13·7	77	2·83	2·47	2·11	75	2·9	6·9

[1]To women married once only.

b. by Regional Health Authority—1974

Regional Health Authority	Total live births (thousands)	Birth rate per 1,000 home population	Total period fertility rates	Illegitimate births (thousands)	Extra-maritally conceived births[1] (thousands)
England and Wales ...	639·9	13·0	1·91	56·5	107·3
Northern ...	39·8	12·7	1·91	3·7	7·9
Yorkshire ...	47·2	13·2	1·98	4·7	8·7
Trent ...	59·0	13·0	1·91	5·0	10·1
East Anglian ...	23·8	13·5	1·97	1·6	3·3
NW Thames ...	45·1	13·0	1·71	4·3	7·1
NE Thames ...	49·9	13·4	1·87	4·8	8·0
SE Thames ...	44·1	12·2	1·83	4·5	7·5
SW Thames ...	33·8	11·7	1·73	2·7	4·6
Wessex ...	34·2	13·0	1·93	2·6	4·9
Oxford ...	30·5	14·0	1·92	1·9	3·6
South Western ...	38·5	12·3	1·91	2·9	5·9
West Midlands ...	70·1	13·5	1·96	5·8	11·2
Mersey ...	32·5	13·0	1·93	3·0	6·3
North Western ...	54·4	13·3	2·02	5·9	11·0
Wales ...	36·2	13·1	1·99	3·0	6·8

Source: OPCS

All figures, whether for hospital region or regional health authority, relate to usual residence of mother.

The total period fertility rate has been derived from summing the fertility rates for five-year age groups up to age 44. It measures the average number of live-born children which would result if women experienced these prevailing rates as they passed through their reproductive period.

The fertility rate for a given period for a given age group is the number of children born to women of that age group in that period divided by the total number of women of that age.

[1] Includes births to remarried women.

27

LIVE BIRTHS CONCEIVED OUTSIDE MARRIAGE—1963 and 1973
By Hospital Region

Table A.9

England and Wales

Hospital Region	Illegitimate births as a % of all births			Pre-maritally conceived live births as a % of all live births[1][2]			Total extra-maritally conceived live births as a % of all live births			Extra-maritally conceived live births %	Abortions to single, widowed, divorced, separated %
	1963	1973	Index (1963=100)	1963	1973	Index (1963=100)	1963	1973	Index (1963=100)	1973	1973
England and Wales	6·9	8·6	125	7·5	7·7	103	14·5	16·3	112	100	100
Total (thousands) ...	59·1	58·1	—	64·4	52·3	—	123·5	110·4	—	110·4	63·7
Newcastle	5·2	9·0	173	7·5	10·0	133	12·7	19·0	150	7·1	4·5
Leeds	7·3	9·8	136	7·7	8·7	113	15·0	18·5	123	7·5	4·9
Sheffield	6·2	8·6	139	7·8	8·4	108	14·0	17·0	121	10·1	6·9
East Anglian	6·2	6·4	103	7·3	6·5	89	13·5	12·9	96	3·1	2·6
NW Metropolitan	9·4	9·2	98	7·6	6·3	83	17·0	15·5	91	7·9	15·9
NE Metropolitan	7·3	7·8	107	6·6	5·9	89	13·9	13·7	99	5·7	7·1
SE Metropolitan	8·0	8·4	105	7·3	6·0	82	15·4	14·4	94	5·7	7·7
SW Metropolitan	8·6	10·2	119	6·8	6·3	93	15·5	16·6	107	6·3	11·8
Wessex	7·0	7·4	106	6·0	6·4	107	13·1	13·8	105	3·5	3·1
Oxford	6·0	6·1	102	6·6	5·9	89	12·6	12·0	95	3·4	3·7
South Western	6·4	7·7	120	7·2	7·4	103	13·6	15·1	111	5·9	5·4
Birmingham	6·9	8·0	116	7·6	7·5	99	14·5	15·5	107	10·5	10·4
Manchester	7·1	10·4	146	8·3	9·1	110	15·4	19·6	127	11·2	7·7
Liverpool	5·3	9·6	181	8·1	10·6	131	13·4	20·2	151	5·7	4·2
Welsh	4·8	7·6	158	9·4	10·7	114	14·2	18·3	129	6·3	4·2

Source: OPCS

Note: The last two columns show the percentage of total events that occurred in each region.

[1] To women married once only.
[2] Births within 8 months of marriage.

28

THE PERCENTAGE OF LIVE AND STILL BIRTHS TAKING PLACE IN NHS HOSPITALS—1966–1973

By Hospital Region and Type of Hospital—1966 and 1969–1973

Table A.10 — England and Wales

Live Births — Percentage of Regional Live Births

Hospital Region		1966	1969	1970	1971	1972	1973
England and Wales	NHS Hospitals Type A[1]	(72·2)	12·1	11·8	11·7	11·0	9·9
	" B[2]		69·6	72·8	75·5	78·6	82·2
	Non-NHS hospitals	2·6	1·9	1·8	1·8	1·8	1·8
	Domiciliary and others	25·2	16·4	13·6	11·0	8·6	6·1
Newcastle	NHS Hospitals Type A	(72·3)	12·1	11·1	8·1	8·9	9·0
	" B		71·8	76·0	82·4	82·9	84·7
Leeds	NHS Hospitals Type A	(74·1)	10·2	10·2	13·4	12·4	10·1
	" B		74·3	75·9	74·6	77·7	83·2
Sheffield	NHS Hospitals Type A	(65·1)	11·3	11·5	11·3	10·8	10·3
	" B		66·0	69·1	72·7	76·1	79·8
East Anglian	NHS Hospitals Type A	(56·7)	11·7	11·8	12·5	12·2	11·3
	" B		55·4	59·2	62·5	66·3	71·4
NW Metropolitan	NHS Hospitals Type A	(75·6)	2·6	2·2	2·2	2·1	1·7
	" B		80·1	82·8	85·0	87·9	90·0
NE Metropolitan	NHS Hospitals Type A	(73·2)	4·1	4·3	4·0	3·9	5·3
	" B		74·9	77·6	79·5	81·6	83·8
SE Metropolitan	NHS Hospitals Type A	(71·6)	8·0	8·0	8·3	8·1	5·4
	" B		71·3	75·1	77·0	79·8	85·3
SW Metropolitan	NHS Hospitals Type A	(76·4)	9·4	5·3	4·2	4·9	5·3
	" B		75·4	81·2	83·6	84·2	85·2
Wessex	NHS Hospitals Type A	(57·6)	17·3	17·2	20·2	15·9	12·4
	" B		61·8	66·2	66·6	73·9	79·0
Oxford	NHS Hospitals Type A	(72·2)	19·8	19·1	18·8	17·0	14·1
	" B		63·3	66·6	70·3	74·3	80·0
South Western	NHS Hospitals Type A	(74·0)	29·3	29·4	30·8	30·4	28·5
	" B		56·8	59·6	61·2	63·8	67·3
Birmingham	NHS Hospitals Type A	(68·2)	14·4	15·1	13·4	12·4	11·5
	" B		64·3	67·2	72·7	76·8	81·2
Manchester	NHS Hospitals Type A	(74·1)	17·4	16·8	16·8	14·5	12·1
	" B		65·5	69·2	71·4	76·3	80·9
Liverpool	NHS Hospitals Type A	(77·9)	5·1	4·9	3·8	4·1	4·1
	" B		80·6	83·0	85·6	87·7	89·6
Welsh	NHS Hospitals Type A	(81·5)	12·9	12·9	11·7	10·2	9·2
	" B		77·2	79·6	81·8	85·1	87·3

Still Births — Percentage of Regional Still Births

Hospital Region		1966	1969	1970	1971	1972	1973
England and Wales	NHS Hospitals Type A[1]	(89·4)	4·4	4·1	3·1	2·4	2·4
	" B[2]		87·5	89·8	90·4	92·2	92·6
	Non-NHS hospitals	1·4	1·1	0·9	1·2	1·1	1·1
	Domiciliary and others	9·2	7·0	5·2	5·3	4·3	3·9
Newcastle	NHS Hospitals Type A	(88·6)	7·7	5·6	1·8	1·5	1·4
	" B		82·9	88·3	93·1	91·3	92·3
Leeds	NHS Hospitals Type A	(89·7)	5·6	3·0	2·6	3·3	1·3
	" B		85·8	90·8	90·0	91·2	92·3
Sheffield	NHS Hospitals Type A	(87·5)	3·6	2·8	4·0	4·0	3·2
	" B		85·8	91·7	87·5	87·5	91·2
East Anglian	NHS Hospitals Type A	(81·9)	2·8	2·9	1·6	1·9	1·5
	" B		77·5	85·9	85·9	89·2	89·7
NW Metropolitan	NHS Hospitals Type A	(90·4)	4·8	0·4	0·3	—	—
	" B		87·9	92·3	93·7	95·3	95·3
NE Metropolitan	NHS Hospitals Type A	(90·4)	1·6	1·1	0·6	0·5	2·5
	" B		92·7	92·8	91·8	94·3	92·9
SE Metropolitan	NHS Hospitals Type A	(90·1)	2·6	2·9	2·1	1·1	1·4
	" B		89·5	91·6	89·9	94·1	95·1
SW Metropolitan	NHS Hospitals Type A	(87·4)	5·5	3·4	0·6	0·6	2·7
	" B		86·8	90·6	88·8	93·2	91·7
Wessex	NHS Hospitals Type A	(84·0)	4·7	3·6	3·6	3·5	3·5
	" B		86·5	88·8	86·6	88·6	93·7
Oxford	NHS Hospitals Type A	(92·9)	3·5	3·4	2·9	2·3	2·3
	" B		87·0	90·1	90·0	91·4	93·7
South Western	NHS Hospitals Type A	(90·3)	8·5	7·5	10·4	6·6	7·6
	" B		83·0	89·8	85·5	89·2	88·4
Birmingham	NHS Hospitals Type A	(89·3)	5·5	8·0	3·7	2·3	3·5
	" B		85·8	84·3	85·5	89·2	88·4
Manchester	NHS Hospitals Type A	(90·9)	4·9	5·3	3·8	2·5	3·2
	" B		88·4	89·6	90·0	94·4	92·3
Liverpool	NHS Hospitals Type A	(92·9)	1·2	1·4	0·2	1·7	1·0
	" B		92·6	93·6	94·7	93·4	96·0
Welsh	NHS Hospitals Type A	(90·1)	4·7	5·5	4·0	3·4	2·0
	" B		89·0	89·3	91·6	91·5	93·3

Note: The figures do not include births to mothers who are resident outside England and Wales.

[1] Type A = NHS Hospital with GP Maternity Unit only.
[2] Type B = NHS Hospital with Obstetric Units.

Source: DHSS
Welsh Office.

LIVE BIRTHS BY AGE OF MOTHER (15–44)—1964, 1971, 1973 and 1974

Numbers: Rates[1] per 1,000 population

Table A.11

England and Wales

Age group of mother	Numbers (thousands)				Rates[1] per 1,000 home population			
	1964	1971	1973	1974	1964	1971	1973	1974
15–44[2]	876·0	783·2	676·0	639·9	93·0	84·0	71·7	67·5
15–19[3]	76·7	82·6	73·3	68·7	42·7	51·0	43·9	40·4
20–24	276·1	285·7	223·7	208·1	182·1	154·4	131·0	123·4
25–29	270·7	247·2	243·8	235·6	187·7	154·5	135·4	129·8
30–34	153·5	109·6	91·8	89·1	107·6	77·7	63·6	60·3
35–39	75·4	45·2	34·2	30·3	49·8	32·8	24·6	21·6
40–44	22·3	11·9	8·6	7·5	12·9	8·1	6·1	5·4

Source: OPCS

[1] Rates for women within age band.
[2] Includes births to women under 15 and over 45 years of age.
[3] Includes births to women under 15 years of age.

31

HIGH PARITY BIRTHS[1]—1963, 1971 and 1973
By Hospital Region

Table A.12

England and Wales

Hospital Region	Number of previous liveborn children 4 or more (thousands)			Fifth and higher order births as a percentage of all births			Index 1963=100	
	1963	1971	1973	1963	1971	1973	1971	1973
England and Wales	68·1	35·6	22·7	8·6	5·0	3·7	52	33
Newcastle	5·9	2·1	1·2	11·1	4·7	3·2	36	20
Leeds	4·9	3·0	2·0	9·3	6·3	5·0	62	42
Sheffield	7·0	3·8	2·4	9·0	5·4	4·0	54	34
East Anglia	1·8	0·9	0·7	7·2	3·5	2·7	51	37
NW Metropolitan	4·5	2·6	1·5	6·3	4·3	3·0	57	34
NE Metropolitan	3·8	2·1	1·4	6·9	4·2	3·3	54	37
SE Metropolitan	3·9	1·8	1·1	7·2	3·8	2·6	45	27
SW Metropolitan	3·3	1·8	1·1	6·5	4·2	2·9	55	33
Wessex	2·3	1·0	0·6	7·5	3·5	2·2	45	26
Oxford	2·6	1·3	0·9	8·1	4·1	2·9	51	33
South Western	3·6	1·4	0·9	7·7	3·2	2·3	39	25
Birmingham	8·7	5·6	3·8	10·0	6·9	5·5	65	43
Manchester	6·7	4·0	2·7	8·9	5·9	4·7	60	40
Liverpool	5·1	2·3	1·4	12·1	6·7	4·9	46	27
Welsh	4·1	1·7	1·8	9·3	4·4	3·4	42	28

Source: OPCS

[1] Fifth or higher order legitimate births occurring to married women with at least four liveborn children.

LIVE BIRTHS BY BIRTHPLACE OF MOTHER—1969–1974

Table A.13

England and Wales

Birthplace of mother	Number (thousands)						Percentage of all live births					
	1969¹	1970	1971	1972	1973	1974	1969¹	1970	1971	1972	1973	1974
Total	783·7	784·5	783·2	725·4	676·0	639·9	100·0	100·0	100·0	100·0	100·0	100·0
United Kingdom²	681·3	684·5	689·7	640·0	596·9	564·2	86·9	87·3	88·1	88·2	88·3	88·2
Total outside United Kingdom	91·8	91·5	88·8	83·0	77·5	74·5	11·7	11·7	11·3	11·4	11·5	11·6
Irish Republic³	24·2	23·5	21·6	18·9	16·4	14·6	3·1	3·0	2·8	2·6	2·4	2·3
Australia, Canada, New Zealand	2·2	2·3	2·4	2·4	2·4	2·3	0·3	0·3	0·3	0·3	0·4	0·4
New Commonwealth⁴	46·1	46·0	45·2	43·0	34·1	33·1	5·9	5·9	5·8	5·9	5·1	5·2
Bangladesh, India, Pakistan⁴	20·6	21·3	21·6	21·2	13·6	13·2	2·6	2·7	2·8	2·9	2·0	2·1
Africa	4·9	4·9	5·0	5·1	5·5	5·7	0·6	0·6	0·6	0·7	0·8	0·9
West Indies⁵	15·1	14·1	12·5	10·8	9·1	8·1	1·9	1·8	1·6	1·5	1·3	1·3
Malta, Gibraltar, Cyprus	3·0	3·0	3·1	2·9	2·7	2·8	0·4	0·4	0·4	0·4	0·4	0·4
Remainder of New Commonwealth	2·5	2·6	3·0	3·0	3·2	3·2	0·3	0·3	0·4	0·4	0·5	0·5
Pakistan⁴	·	·	·	·	6·8	6·8	·	·	·	·	1·0	1·1
Other Foreign	19·4	19·7	19·6	18·6	17·7	17·6	2·5	2·5	2·5	2·6	2·6	2·7
Not stated	10·6	8·5	4·6	2·5	1·6	1·2	1·4	1·1	0·6	0·3	0·2	0·2

Source: OPCS

¹Figures relate to April 1969 to March 1970, the first 12 month period for which information is available.
²Including Isle of Man and Channel Isles.
³Including Ireland, part not stated.
⁴Pakistan is included in the New Commonwealth before 1973.
⁵Including Guyana and Belize (formerly British Honduras).

LIVE BIRTHS

ANALYSIS BY COUNTRY OF BIRTH OF MOTHER AND BY REGIONAL HEALTH AUTHORITY OF RESIDENCE OF MOTHER—1974

Table A.14

England and Wales

Country of birth of mother	England and Wales[5]	Northern	Yorkshire	Trent	East Anglian	NW Thames	NE Thames	SE Thames	SW Thames	Wessex	Oxford	South Western	West Midlands	Mersey	North Western	Wales
	Regional Health Authority of residence of mother															
	NUMBERS															
Irish Republic[1]	14,570	160	586	614	226	2,945	2,073	1,112	991	396	699	378	1,945	464	1,677	304
Australia, Canada and New Zealand ...	2,329	61	78	90	105	406	243	238	315	139	191	141	118	55	77	72
New Commonwealth[2]:—	33,122	346	1,633	2,186	407	5,954	6,118	3,562	2,256	737	1,188	658	5,408	331	1,999	339
India	12,297	164	890	1,022	111	2,295	1,204	697	498	226	432	142	3,336	82	1,088	110
Bangladesh	943	11	76	28	7	106	315	43	36	13	26	7	175	10	78	12
Africa	5,725	52	207	483	68	1,283	1,088	740	533	90	192	107	459	68	300	55
West Indies[3]	8,138	16	279	387	86	1,419	1,793	1,362	718	88	316	172	1,119	43	296	44
Malta, Gibraltar and Cyprus	2,777	17	71	89	49	284	1,166	370	155	138	65	85	117	41	85	45
Remainder	3,242	86	110	177	86	567	552	350	316	182	157	145	202	87	152	73
Pakistan	6,840	154	1,421	458	71	565	616	116	223	40	334	73	1,557	34	1,093	85
Other foreign	17,442	352	620	737	1,254	3,707	2,222	1,362	1,826	931	1,331	679	857	381	762	421
Total with mother born outside United Kingdom	74,303	1,073	4,338	4,085	2,063	13,577	11,272	6,390	5,611	2,243	3,743	1,929	9,885	1,265	5,608	1,221
United Kingdom[4]	563,836	38,683	42,810	54,846	21,698	31,526	38,518	37,699	28,121	31,919	26,724	36,503	59,972	31,176	48,725	34,916
Not stated	1,220	94	79	101	55	42	90	53	71	46	31	64	258	74	93	69
Total	639,359	39,850	47,227	59,032	23,816	45,145	49,880	44,142	33,803	34,208	30,498	38,496	70,115	32,515	54,426	36,206
	PERCENTAGES															
Irish Republic[1]...	2·3	0·4	1·2	1·0	0·9	6·5	4·2	2·5	2·9	1·2	2·3	1·0	2·8	1·4	3·1	0·8
Australia, Canada and New Zealand ...	0·4	0·2	0·2	0·2	0·4	0·9	0·5	0·5	0·9	0·4	0·6	0·4	0·2	0·2	0·1	0·2
New Commonwealth[2]:—	5·2	0·9	3·5	3·7	1·7	13·2	12·3	8·1	6·7	2·2	3·9	1·7	7·7	1·0	3·7	0·9
India	1·9	0·4	1·9	1·7	0·5	5·1	2·4	1·6	1·5	0·7	1·4	0·4	4·8	0·3	2·0	0·3
Bangladesh	0·1	0·0	0·2	0·0	0·0	0·2	0·6	0·1	0·1	0·0	0·1	0·0	0·2	0·0	0·1	0·0
Africa	0·9	0·1	0·4	0·8	0·3	2·8	2·2	1·7	1·6	0·3	0·6	0·3	0·7	0·2	0·6	0·2
West Indies[3]	1·3	0·0	0·6	0·7	0·4	3·1	3·6	3·1	2·1	0·3	1·0	0·4	1·6	0·1	0·5	0·1
Malta, Gibraltar and Cyprus	0·4	0·0	0·2	0·2	0·2	0·6	2·3	0·8	0·5	0·4	0·2	0·2	0·2	0·1	0·2	0·1
Remainder	0·5	0·2	0·2	0·3	0·4	1·3	1·1	0·8	0·9	0·5	0·5	0·4	0·3	0·3	0·3	0·2
Pakistan	1·1	0·4	3·0	0·8	0·3	1·3	1·2	0·3	0·7	0·1	1·1	0·2	2·2	0·1	2·0	0·2
Other foreign	2·7	0·9	1·3	1·2	5·3	8·2	4·5	3·1	5·4	2·7	4·4	1·8	1·2	1·2	1·4	1·2
Total with mother born outside United Kingdom	11·6	2·7	9·2	6·9	8·7	30·1	22·6	14·5	16·6	6·6	12·3	5·0	14·1	3·9	10·3	3·4
United Kingdom[4]	88·2	97·1	90·6	92·9	91·1	69·8	77·2	85·4	83·2	93·3	87·6	94·8	85·5	95·9	89·5	96·4
Not stated	0·2	0·2	0·2	0·2	0·2	0·1	0·2	0·1	0·2	0·1	0·1	0·2	0·4	0·2	0·2	0·2
Total	100·0	100·0	100·0	100·0	100·0	100·0	100·0	100·0	100·0	100·0	100·0	100·0	100·0	100·0	100·0	100·0

[1].Includes Ireland, part not stated.
[2].Excluding Pakistan.
[3].Includes Guyana and Belize (formerly British Honduras).
[4].Includes Isle of Man and Channel Isles.
[5].Excludes 526 births to mothers resident outside England and Wales.

Source: OPCS

LIVE AND STILL BIRTHS TO FEMALES AGED 11-19—1961, 1966, 1971 and 1974
by single years of age and age groups
Numbers: Rate per 1,000 females at each age

Table A.15

England and Wales

Age of mother	1961 Live births	1961 Still births	1961 Total births Rate per 1,000	1966 Live births	1966 Still births	1966 Total births Rate per 1,000	1971 Live births	1971 Still births	1971 Total births Rate per 1,000	1974 Live births	1974 Still births	1974 Total births Rate per 1,000
(a) All births												
16	3,740	71	11·54	4,687	85	14·17	5,847	80	18·69	5,542	73	16·02
17	10,272	179	31·89	13,544	195	39·05	15,462	233	47·91	13,910	169	41·30
18	18,252	316	58·28	25,790	353	68·69	25,721	299	79·62	20,704	283	63·50
19	26,645	472	92·77	41,448	570	101·25	34,097	426	106·82	26,999	298	84·69
11-15	877	13	0·49	1,277	26	0·82	1,514	33	0·90	1,569	32	0·86
16-19	58,909	1,038	47·24	85,469	1,203	58·40	81,127	1,038	63·46	67,155	823	50·57
11-19	59,786	1,051	19·76	86,746	1,229	28·58	82,641	1,071	27·73	68,724	855	21·68
(b) Illegitimate												
16	1,621	29	5·04	2,456	43	7·40	2,939	39	9·50	3,147	42	9·20
17	2,597	56	8·41	4,416	73	13·10	5,286	101	17·29	5,262	84	16·38
18	3,265	78	11·66	5,710	103	16·65	5,948	67	21·17	5,616	90	19·70
19	3,542	79	15·57	6,723	115	20·83	5,869	109	24·40	5,283	60	21·52
11-15	871	13	0·49	1,277	26	0·82	1,513	33	0·90	1,553	32	0·85
16-19	11,025	242	9·69	19,305	334	14·46	20,042	316	17·64	19,308	276	16·17
11-19	11,896	255	4·09	20,582	360	7·11	21,555	349	7·61	20,861	308	6·88

Source: OPCS

ABORTIONS TO FEMALES AGED 11–19—1968[1]–1974

Numbers: Rates per 1,000 females at each age: by single years of age and age groups

Table A.16

Residents of England and Wales

Year	11	12	13	14	15	16	17	18	19	11–15	16–19	11–19
						NUMBERS						
1968[1] ...	3	6	21	150	363	559	693	945	1,088	543	3,285	3,828
1969 ...	2	7	38	279	848	1,445	1,816	2,255	2,543	1,174	8,059	9,233
1970 ...	3	20	85	391	1,233	2,530	3,188	3,864	3,936	1,732	13,518	15,250
1971 ...	3	16	77	529	1,671	3,465	4,426	5,193	5,092	2,296	18,176	20,472
1972 ...	—	7	98	586	2,113	4,318	5,395	6,038	6,035	2,804	21,786	24,590
1973[2] ...	4	14	108	693	2,270	5,082	5,775	6,374	6,249	3,089	23,480	26,569
1974[3] ...	1	9	117	718	2,490	5,348	6,225	6,564	6,060	3,335	24,197	27,532
				RATES PER 1,000 FEMALES AT EACH AGE								
1968[1] ...	0·01	0·02	0·07	0·47	1·13	1·76	2·12	2·77	3·03	0·34	2·44	1·30
1969 ...	0·01	0·02	0·12	0·89	2·63	4·49	5·73	6·80	7·36	0·72	6·12	3·13
1970 ...	0·01	0·06	0·26	1·22	3·88	7·76	9·83	12·08	11·80	1·04	10·37	5·13
1971 ...	0·01	0·05	0·22	1·57	5·12	10·92	13·52	15·90	15·76	1·33	14·04	6·78
1972 ...	—	0·02	0·28	1·69	6·24	13·15	16·87	18·39	18·39	1·58	16·70	7·99
1973[2] ...	0·01	0·04	0·30	1·96	6·50	14·97	17·55	19·88	18·90	1·69	17·79	8·46
1974[3] ...	—	0·02	0·31	2·00	7·00	15·26	18·27	19·87	18·81	1·75	17·48	8·36

Age

[1] From 27 April 1968, when the Abortion Act 1967 came into force, to 31 December 1968 only.
[2] There was also one girl aged 10 (rate 0·003).
[3] Provisional figures.

Source: OPCS.
Registrar General's Statistical Review
Supplement on Abortion.

Section B

MARRIAGE, FAMILY AND ENVIRONMENT

Marriage and Divorce

Tables B.1–3 illustrate recent trends in marriage and divorce from the official statistics. Table B.1 shows the steady increase in marriage at all ages for women since 1911. The proportion of women aged 15–19 who are married has increased from $3\frac{1}{2}\%$ to nearly 9% since 1946 while for women aged 20–24 the proportion married has increased from 44% in 1946 to 59% in 1973. These changes have been brought about not only by an increase in first marriage rates, illustrated by Table B.2 for both men and women since 1951, but by a fall in the average age of marriage also. There is some evidence in the figures of a levelling out, if not a slight reversal, of these trends since 1970.

The increase in divorce has been more marked than the increase in marriage, as Table B.3 illustrates. Divorce rates rose from 2·6 per 1,000 marriages in 1951 to 4·1 in 1969 and 9·0 in 1974. The particularly rapid increase in divorce since 1971 is due, in part, to the effect of the Divorce Reform Act passed in 1969. Although divorce is increasing, less than 1 % of currently existing marriages ended in this way in 1974; even in the 25–34 age group, where divorce rates are highest, less than 2 % of married people were divorced in the year. The probability of divorce is greatest for women married under 20 years of age. It has been estimated that if 1971 divorce rates continue then 14 % of girls married under 20 would be divorced within 10 years of marriage—and divorce rates have increased by 50 % since then.

Following the rise in divorce there has been a sharp increase in the number of divorced people in the population. Consequently there has been a marked increase in the number of divorced persons remarrying (see Table B.2); however, remarriage rates have remained relatively constant.

Household and family

Tables B.4, 5 and 6 describe the household and family situation of children and are derived from the 1971 census of population. A household is defined as either one person living alone or a group of people living together and benefiting from a common housekeeping. A family is defined as either a married couple with or without their never-married children or a single father or mother with his or her never-married children. Thus a household need not equate with a family although 76·4% of households comprise one family only. (These and other definitions used in tables derived from the census of population are set out more fully on page 44).

Lone parent families are not always recognised in the census because the information obtained about single mothers living with their own parents does not always enable these separate families to be identified; if living alone they *will be* counted as separate families. Because of this and other problems a special estimate of the number of one-parent families was made for the Finer Committee. This is given in Table B.6 and refers to Great Britain as a whole.

The implication is that the figures in Table B.4 for lone parents are under-stated by the omission of unmarried mothers who have been included, mainly, in married-couple type households. This will not affect the number of married-couple households but it will reduce slightly the number of dependent children in them. Table B.4 shows that about 85% of children are found in house-holds that comprise a two-parent nuclear family only—and 5% in house-holds comprising a one-parent family only. The remaining 10% of children live in households which include persons outside the nuclear family; these are mainly relatives but in some cases they are boarders. Table B.5 looks at the position of two-parent families in greater detail and shows that there is a much greater probability of there being non-family members of the household when there is only *one* dependent child.

It should be noted in these tables that a dependent child is one under the age of 15 or one aged 15–25 and in receipt of full-time education. However, a family is classed as a family with children if there is any unmarried child of the marriage living in the household, whether dependent or not.

Economic Activity of Wives

Tables B.7–9 describe the pattern of married women's participation in the labour force as revealed by the population census. Table B.7 shows the recent trend in female economic activity rates for each age group. It will be noticed that since 1951 the rates for married women have increased at all ages but most dramatically for women aged 35–54, which have doubled, and for women aged 55–64 which have more than trebled; there has been a significant but more modest increase in the rates for single, widowed and divorced women also. Further increases in female participation in the labour force are to be expected. There was, of course, a strong demand for labour in the period since 1951 which would in any case have encouraged greater par-ticipation, but the striking feature of the trend is the increased tendency for married women to return to work once their children have reached a certain age. Table B.8 shows economic activity rates for 1971 for wives by both number of children and age of the youngest child. It shows that, for example, 18% of wives aged 25–29 with a child aged 0–4 are economically active compared with 53% for those whose youngest child is 5–9. Nevertheless, some 20% of wives with a child aged under 5 were working full- or part-time. A good deal of married women's employment is part-time. Table B.9 shows that more than half the employed women with a child under 5 were working less than 21 hours a week. The increase in married women's employment since 1951 has been associated with an increase in the availability of part-time employment. It has also been associated, as noted in section A, with a decline in the birth rate, a decrease in average family size and a concentration of child-bearing into a shorter period of a woman's life, suggesting that the pattern in future will be for a growing proportion of women to work full- or part-time leaving the labour force for a few years only to care for pre-school children at home. Comparison with 1961 shows that while the economic activity rate for married women aged 25–34 had increased from 29·5 to 38·4 (an increase of 30%) for those with a child aged 0–4 it had increased from 11·1 to 19·8 (an increase of 78%).

Social Class of Children

Evidence from a variety of sources suggests that health risks to children vary between social classes as defined by the Registrar General (see for example section C, Table 12).

Table B.10, extracted from the 1971 census, shows the number of children by single years of age classified by the social class of the head of the family, ie., the father in the case of a married couple, otherwise the single parent. There is little variation by age but it is noticeable that there is a steady increase with age in the proportion of children in social class II and a steady decrease with age in the proportion in Social Class IIIM; this could well be due to a tendency for a man's occupation to change from manual to non-manual as he and his children get older.

Poverty

Tables B.11–16 are taken from official Social Security Statistics and show the numbers of families receiving certain social security benefits. Table B.11, based on payments of Family Allowances, is of interest mainly to illustrate the decline of the larger family since 1964. Families with six or more dependent children comprised 2·4% of the family allowance payroll in 1964 but by 1974 this had reduced to 1·2%. It should be noted that families with only one dependent child under 19 are excluded from the table. Table B.12 shows that in November 1974 there were 854,000 children under 16 in Great Britain living in families dependent to some extent on supplementary benefit. Of these, more than half were children in fatherless families. Another third were the children of unemployed men, two-thirds of whom had exhausted their entitlement to National Insurance unemployment benefit (this usually happens after a year's benefit has been paid).

Table B.13 draws attention to the fact that the number of fatherless families receiving supplementary benefit has increased steadily since 1970. The number of divorced mothers has increased dramatically, possibly as a result of the increase in divorce following the 1969 Divorce Reform Act which took effect in 1971. There is little evidence that the overall number of one-parent families has changed but there may now be less reluctance on their part to claim supplementary benefit, even for small amounts, than hitherto.

Supplementary Benefit is not payable to families in which the father works full-time, yet such families may be just as poor as those where the head is unemployed or sick. Table B.14 provides information about the number of families receiving Family Income Supplement (FIS), a benefit introduced in 1971 for low-income families where the head worked full-time; there were 81,000 such families in Great Britain in March 1974, half of them one-parent families, and including 158,000 children altogether.

Estimates of the overall numbers of families and children living at, below, and up to 20% above, the relevant supplementary benefit level were quoted in Chapter 1 of the main Report. These are given in greater detail below.

NUMBERS OF FAMILIES AND CHILDREN IN LOW INCOME GROUPS

Table C
Great Britain

Number of:	Income		
	Below SB level	At or below SB level	Below and up to 20% above SB level
	(thousands)	(thousands)	(thousands)
Families			
Two-parent	90	170	290
One-parent	20	280	300
Total	110	450	590
Children in			
Two-parent families	220	450	780
One-parent families ...	40	540	580
Total	260	990	1,370

These estimates are based on the continuous Family Expenditure Survey and are subject to relatively high margins of sampling error—because the number of observed families living below the supplementary benefit level is small.

Sick Parents

Tables B.16–18 set out some relevant data on the probable number of sick parents and their children. Table B.16 gives information on the number of men in Great Britain receiving Invalidity Benefit. Broadly, this is a special benefit paid to those who have been incapable of work because of sickness for six months or more. In May 1974 there were 366,000 men receiving this benefit of whom 21%, ie. 77,000, had dependent children; there were 177,000 dependent children whose fathers were receiving this benefit. Not all of these families would be living at or below their supplementary benefit level, and included in the table above, because in some cases the wives would be working or there would be occupational sick pay from an employer.

Tables B.17–18 reproduce results from the General Household Survey 1973 which provide estimates of the number of adults reporting limiting long-standing illnesses. The results show that about 6% of married men and women in the 15–44 age group are chronically sick by this definition. For the age group 45–64 the rates are higher, 18% for men and 16% for women. Prevalence is higher in semi-skilled and unskilled socio-economic groups and more so for men than women. Nearly one-third of men aged 45–64 employed on unskilled manual work reported some limiting long-standing illness compared with less than 10% of professional workers of the same age group. This will reflect the more stringent demands of certain occupations for healthy employees as well as differences in morbidity due to social class factors.

The Environment

The remaining tables in this section, B.19–24, provide information on environmental factors and changes in them which are considered to be relevant to child health.

Table B.19 shows the extent to which housing amenities have improved since 1951 as revealed by the censuses of population and housing. The proportion of households without the use of a fixed bath and toilet has fallen from 37·0% and 7·9% respectively in 1951 to 8·7% and 1·1% in 1971. The proportion of households sharing such amenities has also declined. Table B.20 shows that the character of local authority housing completed each year has changed since 1968. An increasing proportion of dwellings approved recently are in smaller blocks and at lower densities per acre than in 1968.

Table B.21 provides some information on the number of households who change address in a year. According to the General Household Survey 1973 about 9% of households with children under 16 changed address in the year before interview. Many of these moves would be local and not involve a change of general practitioner—but for others the move would isolate them temporarily from routine health care and put them at greater risk.

Tables B.22 and 23 provide information on the difference between the housing conditions of "coloured" households and "white" households as revealed by the General Household Survey. Whether or not a household is classified as "coloured" depends on the assessment of the head of the household by the survey interviewer. B.22 shows that on the whole, "coloured" households are more likely to live in accommodation below "the bedroom standard", and more likely to live in accommodation lacking or sharing amenities such as bath, water closet or central heating. This is no doubt associated with the greater probability that "coloured" households are living in privately rented, furnished accommodation—and the much lower probability that they live in local authority or new town housing. By contrast, B.23 shows that the socio-economic profile of "coloured" households is broadly similar to that of "white" households; although a smaller proportion of "coloured" household heads are classified as semi-skilled than is the case for "white" households. The proportions classified as "skilled" and "unskilled" respectively are identical. Within "coloured" households there are larger differences to be observed between West Indian heads and others; West Indian heads are much less likely to be professional workers, employers or managers and much more likely to be skilled, semi-skilled manual workers or personal service workers than other "coloured" or "white" heads of household.

Finally, B.24 shows the pattern of variation between the 87,578 enumeration districts in the value of certain census variables and indicates for any measure what the position will be in the worst 15%, 10%, 5% and 1% of districts on the basis of that criterion.

43

DEFINITIONS FOR TABLES

Household

A household in the census is defined as one person living alone or a group of people (who may or may not be related) living at the same address with common housekeeping.

Households for household composition

The census household composition tables analysing families are concerned with the *de jure* concept of households. These are households where the members analysed are the persons recorded as usually resident members of the household. These exclude any persons recorded as present on census night that are visitors and includes persons recorded as absent on census night.

Enumerated Households

The census housing tables analyse enumerated households. These are households with at least one person recorded as present on census night irrespective of whether or not that person is usually resident at that address.

Families

Families are composed from the persons recorded as usually resident members of a household and can be:—

    (i) a married couple with or without never-married child(ren)—including childless married couples.

    (ii) a mother or father together with her or his never-married child(ren).

A family can consist of grandparents and their never-married grandchildren where there are no parents in the household.

"Adopted", "step" and "in-law" relationships have been treated in census coding as blood relationships but foster relationships are not.

Children

Children in families as defined by the census can be of any age or economic position but have to be never-married (ie. single).

Dependent Children

Dependent children are defined as persons aged under 15 or aged 15–24 and in full-time education.

Wives

Wives are the females in married couple families.

Mothers

Mothers are the female parents of dependent children.

44

2	214,097	428,194	82,696	259,118	85,294	1,086
3	90,703	272,109	33,300	192,483	45,906	420
4	32,630	130,520	10,140	98,184	22,016	180
5 or more...	16,588	91,573	3,767	71,028	16,660	118
Total dependent children	1,135,962	1,135,962	182,387	693,878	255,143	4,554
Total families with dependent children	567,584	567,584	108,183	304,199	151,703	3,499

(c) One-family Households without others—

Dependent children in family:

1	197,853	197,853	50,191	67,720	77,459	2,483
2	201,670	403,340	79,480	244,542	78,316	1,002
3	85,232	255,696	31,758	181,335	42,231	372
4	30,690	122,760	9,756	92,616	20,216	172
5 or more...	15,580	86,021	3,624	66,853	15,432	112
Total dependent children	1,065,670	1,065,670	174,809	653,066	233,654	4,141
Total families with dependent children	531,025	531,025	103,645	285,702	138,507	3,171

(c) AS A PERCENTAGE OF (a)

Dependent children in family:

1	89·5	89·5	89·5	90·5	88·6	88·1
2	92·7	92·7	93·9	93·2	90·1	89·8
3	92·8	92·8	93·7	93·2	90·4	84·9
4	92·8	92·8	94·7	93·2	90·2	87·8
5 or more...	92·4	92·4	93·7	92·9	90·3	94·9
Total dependent children	92·1	92·1	92·6	92·9	89·7	88·4
Total families with dependent children	91·5	91·5	91·7	92·5	89·3	88·3

Source: OPCS
Census 1971

For definitions of "household", "families", "children" and "dependent children", see p. 44.

49

MARRIED COUPLES BY NUMBER OF DEPENDENT CHILDREN AND AGE AND ECONOMIC ACTIVITY OF WIFE—1971

England and Wales
10% Sample

Table B.8

Dependent children in family	All ages	AGE OF WIFE								
		Under 20	20–24	25–29	30–34	35–39	40–44	45–49	50–54	55–59
					MARRIED COUPLES—SAMPLE NUMBERS					
0	615,043	6,748	45,693	26,307	11,338	13,029	32,328	67,305	86,795	100,043
1	221,083	5,381	33,125	32,545	20,138	23,613	35,941	37,100	22,069	8,591
2	217,466	890	20,209	45,618	48,646	43,115	33,428	17,961	6,153	1,210
3	91,875	60	4,413	16,346	25,590	23,601	14,468	5,782	1,405	175
4	33,082	4	783	4,746	9,910	9,837	5,519	1,862	378	38
5 or more	16,857	4	145	1,702	5,155	5,726	3,118	866	132	6
Total couples	1,195,406	13,087	104,368	127,264	120,777	118,921	124,802	130,876	116,932	110,063
Total dependent children	1,157,039	7,377	90,669	200,851	262,302	251,793	185,700	102,619	40,810	11,725
				PERCENTAGE OF COUPLES WITH WIFE ECONOMICALLY ACTIVE						
0	44·76	67·77	84·16	82·47	78·55	76·05	72·08	65·08	56·42	45·01
1	42·41	14·35	18·88	25·64	42·26	56·95	59·04	54·99	49·24	39·93
2	38·36	8·20	13·48	23·65	38·75	50·27	51·71	48·43	45·52	40·17
3	34·85	6·67	10·24	20·71	33·69	43·23	43·32	42·46	39·93	37·71
4	31·13	25·00	9·07	16·88	29·90	36·27	37·04	36·90	39·42	39·47
5 or more	26·63	—	7·59	13·63	25·06	30·67	28·42	31·41	30·30	—
Total couples	41·77	41·44	45·96	35·55	40·69	50·92	56·89	58·31	54·21	44·54
Total dependent children	36·49	12·66	14·78	22·16	34·66	44·16	47·18	48·12	46·47	39·74

Age of youngest dependent child

MARRIED COUPLES¹—SAMPLE NUMBERS

Age of youngest dependent child										
All ages	570,290	6,338	58,675	100,954	109,435	105,838	91,494	60,696	26,946	7,876
0–4	267,159	6,320	57,415	86,402	62,586	33,930	15,134	3,715	850	472
5–10	179,806	*	1,223	14,367	42,879	52,516	40,175	21,460	5,854	814
11–15	101,263	*	34	178	3,936	18,379	31,384	27,790	14,727	4,088
16–18	22,062	—	*	*	34	1,013	4,801	7,731	5,515	2,502

PERCENTAGE OF COUPLES WITH WIFE ECONOMICALLY ACTIVE

Age of youngest dependent child										
All ages	38·36	13·41	16·21	23·32	36·77	47·82	51·37	50·63	47·38	39·58
0–4	19·64	13·34	15·39	18·27	22·03	24·09	23·87	26·49	31·53	27·54
5–10	51·28	*	53·80	53·16	54·83	54·46	49·25	43·36	40·93	29·61
11–15	60·57	*	*	68·54	73·96	71·04	64·57	56·93	49·62	41·51
16–18	57·72	—	—	*	82·35	77·10	69·53	59·76	50·70	41·93
1961 0–4	11·4	11·3	11·9	11·1	11·1	11·4	12·2	13·0	18·4	13·7

*Based on fewer than 20 cases

¹ Married couples in this part of the table are restricted to those with at least one dependent child under 19 years of age.

For definitions of "dependent children" and "wives", see p. 44.

Source: OPCS
Census 1971

WIVES AND MOTHERS BY ECONOMIC ACTIVITY, HOURS WORKED, NUMBER AND AGE OF DEPENDENT CHILDREN—1971

Table B.9

England and Wales
10% Sample

	Women with the following number of dependent children						Total women	Total women with dependent children	Total dependent children	Women with dependent children aged:			
	0	1	2	3	4	5 or more				0–4	5–10	11–15	16 and over
(a) All wives and mothers													
Total	669,013	245,571	230,089	97,268	35,198	18,158	1,295,297	626,284	1,238,616	283,304	318,264	240,178	70,128
Economically inactive	376,859	137,487	140,368	63,104	24,248	13,386	755,452	378,593	778,957	225,727	189,213	113,538	31,473
Economically active	292,154	108,084	89,721	34,164	10,950	4,772	539,845	247,691	459,659	57,577	129,051	126,051	38,655
Out of employment	10,954	4,782	3,767	1,625	564	292	21,984	11,030	21,051	4,114	6,034	4,592	943
In employment	281,200	103,302	85,954	32,539	10,386	4,480	517,861	236,661	438,608	53,463	123,017	122,640	37,712
Working the following hours:—													
21 or less	64,009	36,785	39,339	15,455	4,860	2,066	162,514	98,505	192,425	27,389	56,931	48,043	12,981
more than 21	205,007	62,105	43,038	15,542	5,011	2,139	332,842	127,835	226,401	23,082	60,698	69,165	23,111
Not stated	12,184	4,412	3,577	1,542	515	275	22,505	10,321	19,782	2,992	5,388	4,840	1,620
(b) Wives in married couples													
Total	615,043	221,083	217,466	91,875	33,082	16,857	1,195,406	580,363	1,157,039	267,159	296,885	221,508	64,410
Economically inactive	339,732	127,313	134,044	59,853	22,782	12,368	696,092	356,360	734,854	214,683	178,179	105,786	29,604
Economically active	275,311	93,770	83,422	32,022	10,300	4,489	499,314	224,003	422,185	52,476	118,706	115,722	34,806
Out of employment	9,935	3,552	3,248	1,419	495	260	18,909	8,974	17,715	3,334	5,109	3,823	795
In employment	265,376	90,218	80,174	30,603	9,805	4,229	480,405	215,029	404,470	49,142	113,597	111,899	34,011
Working the following hours:—													
21 or less	59,803	33,731	37,505	14,704	4,614	1,957	152,314	92,511	181,873	26,164	53,834	45,049	12,162
more than 21	194,062	52,638	39,343	14,453	4,701	2,016	307,213	113,151	204,378	20,232	54,804	62,376	20,407
Not stated	11,511	3,849	3,326	1,446	490	256	20,878	9,367	18,219	2,746	4,959	4,474	1,442

Source: OPCS
Census 1971

For definitions of "dependent children", "wives" and "mothers", see p. 44.

PERSONS IN FAMILIES BY AGE AND BY SOCIAL CLASS OF FAMILY HEAD[1]—1971

Table B.10

England and Wales
10% Sample

Social class of family head	All ages	Age of persons in families												
		0	1	2	3	4	5	6	7	8	9	10–14	15–19	0–19
		SAMPLE NUMBERS												
I Professional, etc., occupations	206,696	4,307	4,223	4,448	4,479	4,560	4,697	4,728	4,645	4,398	4,224	18,106	12,968	75,783
II Intermediate occupations	757,974	11,309	11,292	11,820	12,509	13,234	13,602	14,402	14,260	14,238	14,024	65,815	56,112	252,617
III(N) Skilled occupations–Non-manual	432,216	7,434	7,273	7,407	7,343	7,609	7,380	7,495	7,480	7,062	7,035	32,458	29,658	135,634
III(M) Skilled occupations–Manual	1,500,765	29,366	29,555	30,290	30,370	31,371	31,336	31,287	30,812	30,341	29,088	132,028	112,049	547,893
IV Partly-skilled occupations	679,824	11,393	11,379	11,919	11,451	12,036	12,198	12,463	12,389	12,339	12,258	57,860	54,447	232,132
V Unskilled occupations	275,547	4,946	5,060	4,877	4,819	4,943	4,929	5,065	4,927	4,989	4,870	22,954	22,268	94,647
Not classified	178,494	2,849	2,640	2,537	2,430	2,573	2,482	2,518	2,507	2,454	2,359	10,480	8,490	44,319
Economically inactive	171,552	3,528	3,412	3,636	3,651	3,726	3,759	3,569	3,627	3,507	3,531	15,677	14,980	66,603
Total	4,203,068	75,132	74,834	76,934	77,052	80,052	80,383	81,527	80,647	79,328	77,389	355,378	310,972	1,449,628
		PERCENTAGES												
I Professional, etc, occupations	4·9	5·7	5·6	5·8	5·8	5·7	5·8	5·8	5·8	5·5	5·5	5·1	4·2	5·2
II Intermediate occupations	18·0	15·1	15·1	15·4	16·2	16·5	16·9	17·7	17·7	17·9	18·1	18·5	18·0	17·4
III(N) Skilled occupations–Non-manual	10·3	9·9	9·7	9·6	9·5	9·5	9·2	9·2	9·3	8·9	9·1	9·1	9·5	9·4
III(M) Skilled occupations–Manual	35·7	39·1	39·5	39·4	39·4	39·2	39·0	38·4	38·2	38·2	37·6	37·2	36·0	37·8
IV Partly-skilled occupations	16·2	15·2	15·2	15·5	14·9	15·0	15·2	15·3	15·4	15·6	15·8	16·3	17·5	16·0
V Unskilled occupations	6·6	6·6	6·8	6·3	6·3	6·2	6·1	6·2	6·1	6·3	6·3	6·5	7·2	6·5
Not classified	4·2	3·8	3·5	3·3	3·2	3·2	3·1	3·1	3·1	3·1	3·0	2·9	2·7	3·1
Economically inactive	4·1	4·7	4·6	4·7	4·7	4·7	4·7	4·4	4·5	4·4	4·6	4·4	4·8	4·6

Source: OPCS
Census 1971

[1] Family heads are taken as the husband in married couple families and the lone parent in lone parent families

FAMILIES RECEIVING FAMILY ALLOWANCE AT 31 DECEMBER

Analysis by size of family with total number of children—1964–1974

Table B.11

England and Wales

	Units	1964	1965	1966	1967	1968	1969	1970	1971	1972	1973	1974
Total number of children in families receiving allowances ...	Thousands	8,951	9,154	9,354	9,579	9,782	9,905	10,008	10,133	10,156	10,339	10,263
Number of children attracting allowances	Thousands	5,561	5,695	5,823	5,960	6,083	6,148	6,195	6,248	6,233	6,330	6,241
Number of families receiving allowances:												
All families	Thousands Per cent	3,389 100·0	3,459 100·0	3,531 100·0	3,618 100·0	3,699 100·0	3,757 100·0	3,813 100·0	3,884 100·0	3,924 100·0	4,008 100·0	4,022 100·0
With 2 children	Thousands Per cent	2,050 60·5	2,080 60·1	2,112 59·8	2,160 59·7	2,205 59·6	2,240 59·6	2,284 59·9	2,346 60·4	2,399 61·1	2,470 61·6	2,525 62·8
With 3 children	Thousands Per cent	835 24·6	853 24·7	881 24·9	905 25·0	932 25·2	959 25·5	975 25·6	992 25·5	996 25·4	1,008 25·2	996 24·8
With 4 children	Thousands Per cent	308 9·1	326 9·4	335 9·5	349 9·6	356 9·6	357 9·5	360 9·5	363 9·3	357 9·1	358 8·9	347 8·6
With 5 children	Thousands Per cent	116 3·4	119 3·4	122 3·5	123 3·4	126 3·4	126 3·3	122 3·2	120 3·1	115 2·9	115 2·9	107 2·6
With 6 or more children ...	Thousands Per cent	80 2·4	81 2·3	81 2·3	81 2·2	86 2·2	75 2·0	71 1·9	64 1·6	57 1·5	56 1·4	47 1·2

Source: DHSS
4% Sample

56

SUPPLEMENTARY BENEFIT

Numbers receiving regular weekly payments on 5 November 1974; Recipients and Dependants

Table B.12

Great Britain
Thousands

	All supplementary benefits	Supplementary pensions			Supplementary allowances							
		All pensions	Retirement pensioners and NI widows aged 60 and over	Others	All allowances	Unemployed		Sick and disabled		NI widows under age 60	Women with dependent children	Others
						With NI benefit	Without NI benefit	With NI benefit	Without NI benefit			
Number of persons provided for	4,092	2,136	2,036	101	1,955	212	514	184	201	62	728	53
Persons in receipt of regular weekly payments	2,680	1,807	1,712	96	872	73	228	95	165	42	245	24
Number of dependants:												
Wives	538	322	318	4	216	44	99	54	13	..		6
Total children under 16 years	854	5	5	—	849	94	183	34	22	19	475	22
Under 5 years	264	—	—	—	264	36	52	7	5	1	158	5
5–10 years	338	2	2	—	336	35	71	12	9	4	196	9
11–12 years	106	1	1	—	105	10	25	5	3	4	55	3
13–15 years	145	2	2	—	143	13	34	11	5	10	67	4
Other dependants 16 years and over	20	2	2	—	18	2	3	2	1	2	8	—

Source: DHSS; Samples of 1 in 160 supplementary pension cases and 1 in 40 supplementary allowance cases.

SUPPLEMENTARY BENEFIT

Recipients of regular weekly payments on a day in November 1970–1974

One–parent families

Table B.13

England and Wales
Thousands

| | Total one-parent families | Families headed by a man | Families headed by a woman | Situation of woman | | | | |
				Single	Widowed	Divorced	Prisoner's wife	Separated
1970	195	5	189	51	22	31	7	78
1971	219	6	213	56	23	37	6	91
1972	230	6	224	57	23	42	5	97
1973	231	6	225	57	21	50	5	92
1974	242	7	235	63	16	59	4	94

Source: DHSS; Samples of 1 in 160 supplementary pension cases and 1 in 40 supplementary allowance cases.

FAMILY INCOME SUPPLEMENT

Number[1] of families in receipt of Family Income Supplement, analysed by family type and size at 26 March 1974

Table B.14   Great Britain

Family type	Number of children in family								
	All	1	2	3	4	5	6	7	8 or more
NUMBERS									
Two-parent families	39,874	7,082	9,666	8,882	6,949	3,775	2,015	804	702
One-parent families headed by a man ...	1,068	305	356	407				—	—
One-parent families headed by a woman ...	40,057	24,684	9,350	6,023				—	—
All families	81,000	32,070	19,372	12,881	8,598	4,385	2,188	804	702
INDICES (1972=100)[2]									
Two-parent families	68	54	63	71	77	77	81	70	105
One-parent families headed by a man ...	70	55	115	61				—	—
One-parent families headed by a woman ...	140	125	156	204				—	—
All families	91	98	90	86	85	84	84	69	105

Source: DHSS.

[1] Based on a 10% sample of claims 1974.
[2] Earliest comparison 1972: based on a 20% sample as at 25 April 1972.

MALES RECEIVING UNEMPLOYMENT BENEFIT ON THE FIRST MONDAY IN MAY AND NOVEMBER, ANALYSED BY DEPENDENCY CONDITION AND WHETHER RECEIVING SUPPLEMENTARY ALLOWANCE—1968-1974

Table B.15

Great Britain

Thousands

	1968		1969		1970		1971		1972		1973		1974	
	May	Nov.	May	Nov.	May	Nov.	May	Nov.	May	Nov.	May	Nov.	May	Nov.
All males	264	255	246	242	263	260	343	393	389	293	212	166	202	234
with supplementary allowance	64	55	59	58	60	54	87	98	104	76	52	38	54	60
without supplementary allowance	200	200	187	184	203	206	256	295	285	217	160	138	148	173
No dependants	114	110	105	108	115	120	160	191	181	140	98	75	91	113
with supplementary allowance	21	15	16	18	18	17	27	33	37	29	19	13	19	22
without supplementary allowance	93	95	89	90	97	104	133	158	144	111	79	62	72	91
Adult dependant only	51	54	51	47	52	51	57	62	65	54	45	38	38	40
with supplementary allowance	8	8	8	8	8	8	10	10	11	8	6	5	5	5
without supplementary allowance	43	46	43	39	44	43	47	52	54	46	39	33	33	35
Adult dependant and child(ren)	80	74	71	69	77	68	99	110	110	76	53	42	55	60
with supplementary allowance	32	30	30	29	31	27	45	49	50	35	24	19	27	30
without supplementary allowance	48	44	41	39	46	42	54	61	60	41	29	23	28	30
Child dependant(s) only	19	18	18	18	19	20	27	31	33	23	16	12	18	21
with supplementary allowance	3	3	4	3	3	3	5	5	5	4	3	2	3	4
without supplementary allowance	15	15	15	15	16	17	22	25	27	19	13	11	15	17
Average number of children for males with child dependants	2·5	2·5	2·5	2·5	2·5	2·4	2·4	2·4	2·4	2·3	2·4	2·4	2·4	2·4
with supplementary allowance	2·7	2·8	2·8	2·8	2·7	2·7	2·7	2·7	2·7	2·6	2·7	2·7	2·7	2·7
without supplementary allowance	2·5	2·4	2·3	2·3	2·4	2·3	2·2	2·2	2·2	2·1	2·2	2·2	2·2	2·2

Source: Department of Employment
5% sample of cases

NUMBERS OF INCAPACITATED MALES IN RECEIPT OF INVALIDITY BENEFIT AND PROPORTION IN RECEIPT OF AN INCREASE IN RESPECT OF CHILD DEPENDANTS WITH AVERAGE NUMBER OF DEPENDENT CHILDREN PER FATHER—1972–1974

Table B.16   Great Britain

Age of beneficiary at 31 May	June		
	1972	1973	1974
Number of beneficiaries:			
All ages	334	355	366
Under 20	—	—	—
20–24	4	3	3
25–29	7	8	7
30–34	8	9	11
35–39	12	13	14
40–44	17	19	20
45–49	29	29	30
50–54	41	47	50
55–59	65	66	65
60–64	139	146	148
65–69	12	14	17
Percentage with child dependants:			
All ages	19	19	21
Under 20	—	67	—
20–24	28	33	31
25–29	38	43	48
30–34	55	51	51
35–39	59	61	65
40–44	54	52	58
45–49	41	43	44
50–54	28	27	29
55–59	14	14	15
60–64	4	5	5
65–69	3	3	4
Average number of children per father:			
All ages	2·2	2·3	2·3
Under 20	—	1·0	—
20–24	1·4	1·8	1·7
25–29	2·4	2·5	2·3
30–34	2·8	2·9	3·0
35–39	3·2	3·2	3·2
40–44	2·9	2·8	2·8
45–49	2·4	2·4	2·3
50–54	1·8	1·9	1·9
55–59	1·5	1·5	1·6
60–64	1·3	1·4	1·4
65–69	1·3	1·2	1·3

Source: DHSS
2½% sample of cases

CHRONIC SICKNESS: PERSONS AGED 15 OR OVER REPORTING LIMITING LONG-STANDING ILLNESS BY SEX, AGE AND MARITAL STATUS—1973

(a) Rates per 1,000

(b) Standardised for age: observed rates as % of expected rates[1]

Table B.17   Great Britain

Marital Status	(a) Males				(a) Females				(b) Males	(b) Females
	Total	15–44	45–64	65+	Total	15–44	45–64	65+		
Single ⋮ ⋮ ⋮	79	55	210	320	114	51	233	353	96	102
Married ⋮ ⋮ ⋮	153	63	183	352	124	58	155	329	100	93
Widowed/divorced/separated ⋮	268	48[2]	267	336	302	119	256	360	105	112
Rate for all persons in each sex/age group ⋮ ⋮ ⋮	143	60	189	346	154	59	177	348	100	100

[1] Great Britain = 100.
[2] Based on 10 or fewer observations.

Source: OPCS
General Household Survey

CHRONIC SICKNESS: PERSONS REPORTING LIMITING LONG-STANDING ILLNESS BY SEX, AGE AND SOCIO-ECONOMIC GROUP—1973

Rates per 1,000

Table B.18   Great Britain

| | Rates per 1,000 | | | | | |
| | Males | | | Females | | |
Socio-economic Group[1]	15–44	45–64	65+	15–44	45–64	65+
Professional	33	93	[14][2]	28[3]	131	[10][2]
Employers and managers	53	117	311	53	111	293
Intermediate and junior non-manual	66	194	365	49	179	358
Skilled manual (incl. foremen and supervisors) and own account non-professional	52	197	375	57	175	367
Semi-skilled manual and personal service	67	235	339	71	204	349
Unskilled manual	94	326	333	90	237	323
Rate for all persons in each sex/age group	60	189	346	59	177	348

Source: OPCS
General Household Survey

[1] Members of the armed forces, inadequately described occupations and all persons (including students) who have never worked, have not been shown as separate categories but are included in the rates for all persons.
[2] The number of observations only is shown [bracketed] where the base figure is less than 100.
[3] Based on 10 or fewer observations.

HOUSING AMENITIES—1951–1971

Percentage of households lacking or sharing amenities

Table B.19   England and Wales

	1951	1961	1966	1971
Percentage of all households[1] entirely without certain amenities—				
Fixed bath	37·0	22·0	15·0	8·7
Water Closet:				
Internal or external ...	7·9	6·9	1·8	1·1
Internal	..	..	19·8	12·1
Hot water tap	..	21·9	12·5	6·4
Percentage of all households sharing certain amenities—				
Fixed bath	7·6	4·6	4·3	3·4
Water Closet:				
Internal or external ...	13·4	5·8	6·0	4·0
Internal	..	..	4·1	3·3
Hot water tap	..	1·8	2·1	2·0

[1] In permanent and non-permanent buildings.
For definitions of "households", see p. 44.

Source: OPCS
Census of Population

LOCAL AUTHORITY HOUSING: STOREY HEIGHT AND DENSITY—1968–1973

Table B.20

England and Wales
Percentages

		1968	1969	1970	1971	1972	1973
Storey heights							
Houses:	1 storey	7·4	9·7	9·1	10·0	9·8	11·4
	2 or 3 storeys ...	41·9	40·8	42·4	40·0	38·7	43·9
Flats:	2 to 4 storeys	30·8	35·9	38·6	41·4	44·1	41·7
	5 to 9 storeys	10·5	8·0	7·2	5·2	5·4	2·3
	10 to 14 storeys ...	3·5	1·8	1·0	1·5	0·7	0·2
	15 or more storeys ...	5·9	3·8	1·7	1·9	1·3	0·5
Density of persons per acre							
Under 60·0		25·8	37·0	35·0	38·1	34·5	39·1
60·0 to 79·9		36·7	30·1	34·0	30·1	32·9	41·0
80·0 to 99·9		12·6	9·6	11·2	14·8	12·5	9·5
100·0 to 139·9		9·9	9·5	12·5	9·1	10·2	6·3
140·0 to 199·9		9·4	10·8	5·7	5·2	8·1	3·1
200·0 or more		5·6	3·0	1·6	2·7	1·8	1·0
Average number of persons per acre		*71·2*	*66·4*	*65·2*	*63·3*	*65·3*	*61·0*

Source: Department of the Environment
Housing and Construction Statistics

PEOPLE WHO MOVED HOUSEHOLD IN PREVIOUS TWELVE MONTHS—1973

Table B.21

	Heads of household who moved in past year			Heads of household who did not move in past year	All households in sample (= 100%)
	Continuing[1] HOH	New[1] HOH	All HOHs		
Percentage of each household type:					
Households:					
With children under 16 ...	7·2	2·1	9·4	90·6	3,852
Without children under 16:					
One person aged 16–59	9·0	7·5	16·5	83·5	636
One person aged over 60	2·2	0·2	2·4	97·6	1,568
Two persons aged 16–59	6·8	8·3	15·1	84·9	1,645
Two persons at least one aged over 60	2·2	0·4	2·6	97·4	2,008
Three persons or more ...	3·0	0·9	3·9	96·1	1,929
All household types	5·0	2·5	7·6	92·4	11,638

Source: OPCS

General Household Survey

[1]The head of household (HOH) is "continuing" if he/she was also head of the household he/she moved from; if not, the HOH is "new".

COLOUR OF HEAD OF HOUSEHOLD BY BEDROOM STANDARD, AMENITIES AND TENURE—1971–1973 combined

Table B.22   Great Britain

| | Colour of Head of Household[1] | | | |
| | White | | Coloured | Total |
	UK-born	Other		
	%	%	%	%
Difference from Bedroom Standard:				
Below standard	5	10	25	6
Equals standard	33	39	43	33
Above standard	62	50	32	61
Amenities:				
Bath or Shower:				
Sole use	89	84	71	88
Shared	3	9	19	3
None	8	7	10	9
W.C.:				
Sole use	96	90	79	95
Shared	3	10	21	4
None	1	—	—	1
Central heating:				
Yes	37	40	25	37
No	63	60	75	63
Tenure:				
Owner occupied[2]	49	48	51	49
Rented with job/business	4	4	4	4
Rented from local authority/New Town	32	26	18	32
Rented from housing association ...	1	1	1	1
Rented privately—unfurnished	12	11	8	11
Rented privately—furnished	2	10	18	3
BASE (=100%)	31,446	1,329	656	33,431

Source: OPCS
General Household Survey

[1]1973 estimates for "coloured" and "other white" households are subject to relatively large sampling error. This is reduced substantially if data spread over 3 years are aggregated.

[2]The bedroom standard is assessed by allowing one bedroom for each married couple, one for each other person over 21 and one for each two persons under 21 with the proviso that those aged 10 to 20 should share a bedroom only with a person of the same sex.

[3]A split between outright owners and mortgagors is available only for 1973, viz:

		Outright owners	Mortgagors
UK-born	...	23%	26%
Other white	...	17%	27%
Coloured	...	12%	41%

COLOUR OF HEAD OF HOUSEHOLD BY COUNTRY OF BIRTH AND SOCIO-ECONOMIC GROUP—1971–1973 COMBINED

Table B.23   Great Britain

Interviewer's Assessment of Colour and Country of Birth

Socio-economic Group of Head of Household	White	Coloured				TOTAL
		West Indies	India	Elsewhere	All countries	
Professional	% 4	% 2	% 8	% 8	% 6	% 4
Employers and managers	14	1	8	8	5	14
Intermediate and junior non-manual ...	21	9	20	21	17	21
Skilled manual (including foremen and supervisors) and own account non-professional ...	33	47	35	22	33	33
Semi-skilled manual and personal service ...	19	32	16	22	24	19
Unskilled	7	7	9	6	7	7
Full-time students	—	2	1	10	5	1
Never worked	2	Nil	3	2	2	2
Base (= 100%)	32,609	224	138	183	645	33,254

Source: OPCS
General Household Survey

67

SUMMARY STATISTICS OF FREQUENCY DISTRIBUTIONS OF CENSUS INDICATORS—1971
All Enumeration Districts[1]

Table B.24

Great Britain Percentages

	Mean	Standard deviation	15% cut-off value	10% cut-off value	5% cut-off value	1% cut-off value
Housing						
% of private households who share or lack hot water	9·7	13·6	22·1	28·0	38·2	61·0
% of private households who share or lack bath	14·5	20·0	34·4	44·0	58·8	86·8
% of private households in permanent buildings who lack bath	10·4	18·0	23·8	33·6	50·5	85·9
% of private households who lack inside WC	12·5	19·4	30·3	40·6	57·0	85·2
% of private households living at a density of greater than 1·5 persons per room	2·3	4·5	4·3	6·2	10·1	23·5
% of private households living at a density of greater than 1 person per room	8·1	8·8	14·6	18·3	25·7	43·9
% of private households in shared dwellings	4·7	11·8	7·1	13·4	29·1	62·6
% of private households not having exclusive use of all basic amenities	20·2	23·6	47·2	56·8	71·0	93·2
Employment						
% of economically active males unemployed, but seeking work or sick	5·8	4·9	9·8	11·7	15·1	24·0
% of economically active females unemployed, but seeking work or sick	5·1	4·1	8·6	9·9	12·3	18·9
Assets						
% of private households with no car	53·9	20·1	74·7	78·3	83·4	91·8
Socio-economic group						
% of economically active and retired males in SEG 11 (unskilled manual workers)	8·3	10·0	17·8	21·5	27·8	41·6
Special needs						
% of total population present in private households of age 0–14	23·0	7·4	30·2	32·4	35·7	41·9
Pensioner households (households of 1 or 2 persons with 1 or 2 persons of pensionable age) as % of all private households present	27·2	11·9	38·7	41·7	46·8	59·1
% of population born in New Commonwealth with one or both parents born in New Commonwealth, or born in Great Britain with both parents born in New Commonwealth	3·6	7·4	4·7	8·8	17·4	39·4
Housing tenure						
% of private households in accommodation rented from local authority	31·1	37·9	92·8	97·5	99·3	100·0
% of private households in privately rented unfurnished accommodation	17·5	19·2	36·9	44·8	57·9	83·9
% of private households in privately rented furnished accommodation	5·1	10·4	9·3	14·8	26·4	52·3

[1] 87, 578 Enumeration Districts.
For definitions of "household", see p. 44.

Source: Central Statistical Office (Social Trends No. 6—HMSO, 1975)

Section C

MORTALITY

Tables C.1 and 2 set out recent trends in child mortality in a broad historical context. Infant mortality, which accounted for more than 10% of all births at the beginning of the century, has declined rapidly to the current level of 16 per 1,000 live births and is still declining. It will be noted that the greatest improvement has been due to the prevention of death in the period between 6 months and a year and the least in prevention of first day deaths. However, the extent to which the decline in stillbirth rates has affected this category is unknown.

The following table sets out the improvement in mortality rates since 1951 for children in various age groups—the provisional figures for 1975 confirm that these improvements have been sustained.

SUMMARY OF CHANGES IN INFANT AND CHILD MORTALITY RATES SINCE 1951

Table D

Rate	1951 Rate	1974	
		Rate	Index 1951=100
Infant Mortality rates per 1,000 live births			
Under one year	29·7	16·3	55
Under 1 day	7·5	5·2	69
1 day and under 1 week	8·0	4·2	53
1 week and under 4 weeks	3·3	1·7	52
4 weeks and under 3 months	4·1	2·3	56
3 months and under 6 months	3·6	1·9	53
6 months and under 1 year	3·2	1·1	34
Child Mortality rates per 1,000 population in age group			
1 year and under 5 years	1·35	0·65	48
5 years and under 10	0·55	0·31	56
10 years and under 15	0·47	0·28	60
15 years and under 20	0·76	0·64	84

Infant mortality rates are valuable indicators of the differences between the health status of different countries and of different regions of the same country. Table C.3 sets out infant mortality rates for each Hospital Region of England and Wales for selected years since 1963. It will be noted that there is considerable variation from one part of the country to another and in the extent to which the various rates have improved. Table G.1 includes the latest infant and child mortality rates for the new health authorities. It will be noted that although the infant mortality rate for England and Wales in 1974 was 16·3 it was as high as 25·21 per 1,000 births in Bradford AHA, and over 20 per 1,000 in Leeds, Walsall, Sunderland, Wirral, Manchester, Oldham, Rochdale, Salford, Tameside and Trafford and Lambeth, Southwark and Lewisham; mainly northern industrial areas. By contrast it was below 13 per 1,000 in Norfolk, Barnet, Hillingdon, Ealing, Hammersmith and Hounslow, Kensington, Chelsea and

Westminster, Bromley, West Sussex and Buckinghamshire—all Southern rural or semi-urban areas or, in the case of Kensington, Chelsea and Westminster, with ready access to hospital.

By contrast, Table C.4 compares the recent experience of a number of countries and shows that although rates of infant mortality have declined in England and Wales they have not fallen so rapidly as in other countries such as France, Finland and Japan.

There are pronounced variations in mortality rates when deaths are analysed by birthweight. Tables C.5 and 6 provide statistics obtained from notifications of births to Medical Officers of Health, now Area Medical Officers on this subject. In 1974, the mortality rate on the first day of life of babies weighing 1,500 grammes or less was nearly 300 times that of those weighing over 2,500 grammes; the factors for stillbirth and late-neonatal mortality rates are 66 and 69 respectively. Table C.5 gives changes since 1954 in the number of low weight births by categories, and in their mortality up to the first 28 days of life. Table C.6 gives data for Regional Health Authorities for 1974.

Improvements in mortality over time have been smaller for first day deaths in all low birthweight groups but it is in the lowest weight group that the least improvement is seen. The greatest improvement in first day deaths amongst low weight babies between 1954 and 1974 is seen in babies weighing between 2,001 and 2,250 grammes where there was a 34% reduction in the mortality rate. For deaths after the first day the mortality rate for all groups improved, ranging from over 57% in the 2,000–2,500 grammes group to 40% in the lowest birthweight group.

Tables C.7–11 set out the trends in deaths and death rates for the main categories of the International Classification of Diseases for children of different age groups; 0–1, 1–4, 5–9, 10–14 and 15–19 respectively.

The main causes of infant deaths are those specific to perinatal mortality—a group only recognised in the International Classification of Diseases since 1968. In 1974 these accounted for 44% of all infant deaths. The next most important group was congenital anomalies (24%) followed by diseases of the respiratory system (13%) which includes pneumonia (8%) and acute respiratory infections (4%). Compared with 20 years ago the relative importance of infective and parasitic diseases (3·5%) and its major components enteritis and other diarrhoeal diseases (1·6%) has declined, as has that of pneumonia and diseases of the respiratory system. Clearly it is those diseases affecting the early neonatal period which have declined least ie. congenital anomalies and the specific causes of perinatal mortality.

From the 1–4 age group onwards, accidents are the major cause of death rising from 23% of all deaths in the 1–4 age group to 62% of male deaths and 38% of female deaths in the 15–19 age group. Road accidents are by far the largest single cause of accidental death in these age groups; 34% in the 1–4 group; 63% in the 5–9 group; 55% in the 10–14 group and 70% in the 15–19 group.

Malignant neoplasms remain the second major cause of death in each group except the 1–4 age group (where they account for 11 % of all deaths). Leukaemia accounted for two-thirds of all deaths from malignant neoplasms in these age groups.

In the 1–4 age group, respiratory diseases accounted for 16 % of all deaths in 1974 but the proportion was only 8 % in the 5–9 and 10–14 age groups. The death rate was markedly higher in the 15–19 age group—much more so for boys than girls—but in this age group respiratory diseases accounted for only 6 % of deaths.

Congenital anomalies accounted for 19 % of all deaths in the 1–4 age group, and was the second most important cause of death; but for the 5–9 and 10–14 age groups the death rate is much lower and in 1974 accounted for 13 % and 9 % of deaths respectively, making it the third most important cause of death at these ages.

The main improvement over the past 20 years has come from a great reduction in the death rate for infective and parasitic diseases, pneumonia and other diseases of the respiratory system. These improvements are marked in all age groups. Mortality rates for infective and parasitic diseases are now less than a fifth of what they were in 1951 for the 1–4 age group and the improvement has been even greater for older age groups. Improvements for respiratory diseases have been less dramatic but even so the mortality rate for these has more than halved since 1951 for the 1–4s and 5–9s.

Finally, C.12 shows deaths and death rates from all causes between 1959–63, and from three of the major causes, for children aged 1–14 analysed by the social class of the head of household. With very few exceptions, the rates are highest for social classes IV and V. Equivalent data based on the 1971 census is not yet available but it is expected that, despite the fall in mortality between 1961 and 1971, the social class differences will broadly remain. More recent data on perinatal mortality has just become available which supports this and shows that although perinatal mortality rates have fallen since 1949 for all social classes the social class differences remain and have if anything widened.

PERINATAL MORTALITY RATES: SOCIAL CLASS (LEGITIMATE SINGLE BIRTHS ONLY)—1950 AND 1973

Table E   England and Wales

Social class	1950	1973	Percentage decrease 1950–73
I Professional	25·4	13·9	45
II Managerial	30·4	15·6	49
III Skilled	33·6	19·2	43
non-manual		17·3	
manual		19·7	
IV Semi-skilled	36·9	21·8	41
V Unskilled	40·4	26·8	34
All social classes (including armed forces, students, etc.)	34·9*	18·9	46

* Estimated   Source: OPCS

71

DEATH RATES PER 1,000 POPULATION AGED 1–19 BY SEX AND AGE GROUPS—1901–1974

Table C.1   England and Wales

Period	PERSONS				MALES				FEMALES			
	1–4	5–9	10–14	15–19	1–4	5–9	10–14	15–19	1–4	5–9	10–14	15–19
1901–1905	..	3·74	2·19	3·11	..	3·68	2·14	3·20	..	3·79	2·24	3·02
1906–1910	..	3·38	2·03	2·87	..	3·33	1·97	2·97	..	3·44	2·09	2·76
1911–1915[1]	..	3·39	2·08	2·88	..	3·42	2·05	3·01	..	3·37	2·11	2·75
1916–1920[1]	..	3·81	2·48	3·77	..	3·81	2·41	3·91	..	3·81	2·56	3·66
1921–1925	..	2·48	1·71	2·61	..	2·55	1·69	2·66	..	2·41	1·72	2·56
1926–1930	6·56	2·37	1·57	2·49	6·88	2·48	1·61	2·58	6·23	2·25	1·53	2·41
1931–1935[1]	4·70	2·18	1·41	2·33	5·00	2·28	1·44	2·45	4·40	2·07	1·37	2·22
1936–1940[1]		1·84	1·20	2·01		1·96	1·27	2·15		1·71	1·13	1·87
1941–1945[1]	3·50	1·50	1·08	1·96	3·72	1·69	1·20	2·22	3·26	1·31	0·97	1·74
1946–1950[1]	1·77	0·77	0·62	1·18	1·90	0·88	0·69	1·33	1·62	0·64	0·54	1·05
1951–1955	1·14	0·47	0·41	0·68	1·23	0·55	0·48	0·86	1·04	0·39	0·34	0·50
1956–1960	0·91	0·41	0·34	0·63	0·99	0·49	0·40	0·88	0·82	0·33	0·27	0·38
1961–1965	0·86	0·39	0·33	0·67	0·94	0·47	0·41	0·95	0·78	0·32	0·25	0·38
1966–1970	0·79	0·36	0·32	0·68	0·87	0·43	0·39	0·96	0·70	0·28	0·25	0·39
1951	1·35	0·55	0·47	0·76	1·44	0·65	0·57	0·89	1·26	0·46	0·37	0·64
1952	1·18	0·49	0·43	0·71	1·32	0·57	0·50	0·90	1·03	0·41	0·34	0·52
1953	1·18	0·49	0·41	0·64	1·26	0·56	0·46	0·82	1·09	0·41	0·35	0·46
1954	0·94	0·41	0·37	0·63	1·06	0·48	0·43	0·81	0·82	0·34	0·31	0·46
1955	1·00	0·43	0·38	0·64	1·04	0·49	0·45	0·88	0·97	0·36	0·32	0·40
1956	0·91	0·40	0·34	0·57	0·98	0·46	0·41	0·79	0·83	0·33	0·27	0·36
1957	0·97	0·41	0·38	0·68	1·04	0·48	0·44	0·91	0·90	0·34	0·30	0·45
1958	0·88	0·40	0·32	0·60	0·99	0·49	0·39	0·83	0·77	0·31	0·24	0·35
1959	0·91	0·41	0·34	0·65	1·00	0·49	0·39	0·94	0·81	0·33	0·29	0·37
1960	0·87	0·44	0·32	0·64	0·95	0·53	0·38	0·91	0·78	0·34	0·26	0·36

Year															
1962	…	…	…	0·86	0·38	0·34	0·64	0·94	0·44	0·42	0·92	0·77	0·32	0·25	0·35
1963	…	…	…	0·91	0·40	0·32	0·63	0·98	0·48	0·40	0·90	0·83	0·32	0·24	0·35
1964	…	…	…	0·81	0·39	0·33	0·70	0·87	0·45	0·40	0·99	0·74	0·32	0·25	0·40
1965	…	…	…	0·82	0·39	0·35	0·71	0·87	0·48	0·42	1·01	0·76	0·31	0·29	0·40
1966	…	…	…	0·84	0·37	0·34	0·75	0·92	0·44	0·42	1·08	0·75	0·29	0·25	0·41
1967	…	…	…	0·77	0·37	0·35	0·70	0·84	0·44	0·42	0·99	0·70	0·29	0·27	0·41
1968	…	…	…	0·81	0·37	0·33	0·64	0·88	0·44	0·39	0·89	0·73	0·30	0·26	0·37
1969	…	…	…	0·78	0·34	0·29	0·66	0·89	0·41	0·37	0·92	0·67	0·26	0·21	0·39
1970	…	…	…	0·72	0·33	0·30	0·64	0·80	0·40	0·36	0·92	0·64	0·27	0·23	0·35
1971	…	…	…	0·70	0·37	0·30	0·65	0·77	0·44	0·37	0·90	0·64	0·29	0·24	0·39
1972	…	…	…	0·75	0·35	0·28	0·63	0·78	0·41	0·36	0·86	0·71	0·29	0·20	0·40
1973	…	…	…	0·69	0·33	0·28	0·64	0·77	0·39	0·34	0·86	0·60	0·26	0·21	0·41
1974	…	…	…	0·65	0·31	0·28	0·64	0·72	0·35	0·32	0·89	0·58	0·26	0·23	0·37

Source: OPCS
Registrar General's Statistical Review

[1]Civilian mortality only in 1915–1920, and also from 3 September 1939 to 31 December 1949 for males and from 1 June 1941 to 31 December 1949 for females.

STILLBIRTH RATES AND INFANT DEATH RATES BY AGE—1906 to 1974

Table C.2

England and Wales

Period	Total infant mortality (under 1 year)	Neonatal mortality (under 4 weeks)	Early neonatal mortality (under 1 week)	Late neonatal mortality (1 week and under 4 weeks)	Post-neonatal mortality (4 weeks and under 1 year)	Early neonatal period		Post-neonatal period			Perinatal mortality—Rates per 1,000 total births[2]
						Under 1 day	1 day and under 1 week	4 weeks and under 3 months	3 months and under 6 months	6 months and under 1 year	Stillbirths plus infant deaths under 1 week
1906–1910	117·1	40·2	24·5	15·7	76·9	11·5	13·0	22·8	22·0	32·1	..
1911–1915	108·7	39·0	24·1	14·9	69·8	11·4	12·7	20·2	19·6	30·0	..
1916–1920	90·9	37·0	23·4	13·7	53·9	11·0	12·4	16·5	14·6	22·8	..
1921–1925	74·9	33·4	21·7	11·7	41·6	10·4	11·3	12·8	11·3	17·5	..
1926–1930	67·6	31·8	21·8	9·9	35·7	10·3	11·5	10·8	9·5	15·4	..
1931–1935	61·9	31·4	22·4	9·0	30·5	10·7	11·7	9·9	8·5	12·1	62·5
1936–1940	55·3	29·2	21·5	7·7	26·0	10·4	11·2	8·8	7·8	9·4	59·2
1941–1945	49·8	26·0	18·7	7·2	23·8	9·3	9·5	8·9	7·7	7·2	48·6
1946–1950	36·3	21·1	16·2	4·9	15·2	7·9	8·4	5·8	5·0	4·4	39·8
1951	29·7	18·8	15·5	3·3	10·9	7·5	8·0	4·1	3·6	3·2	38·2
1952	27·6	18·3	15·2	3·2	9·3	7·6	7·6	3·7	3·0	2·6	37·5
1953	26·8	17·7	14·8	2·9	9·1	7·4	7·4	3·4	3·0	2·7	36·9
1954	25·4	17·7	14·9	2·8	7·7	7·6	7·4	3·0	2·6	2·1	38·1
1955	24·9	17·3	14·6	2·6	7·6	7·6	7·0	2·9	2·6	2·1	37·4
1956	23·7	16·8	14·2	2·6	6·9	7·4	6·8	2·7	2·3	1·8	36·7
1957	23·1	16·5	14·1	2·4	6·7	7·6	6·5	2·6	2·1	1·9	36·2
1958	22·5	16·2	13·8	2·4	6·4	7·5	6·3	2·6	2·1	1·7	35·0
1959	22·2	15·9	13·6	2·3	6·3	7·6	6·0	2·4	2·1	1·8	34·1
1960	21·8	15·5	13·3	2·2	6·3	7·5	5·8	2·5	2·1	1·6	32·8

Infant mortality per 1,000 live births[1] at various ages

74

Year											
1962	21·7	15·1	13·0	2·1	6·6	7·4	5·6	2·3	2·3	1·8	30·6
1963	21·1	14·3	12·3	2·0	6·9	7·2	5·1	2·7	2·4	1·8	29·3
1964	19·9	13·8	12·0	1·8	6·1	7·1	4·9	2·4	2·1	1·6	28·2
1965	19·0	13·0	11·3	1·7	6·0	6·6	4·7	2·4	2·1	1·6	26·9
1966	19·0	12·9	11·1	1·7	6·1	6·5	4·6	2·5	2·0	1·6	26·3
1967	18·3	12·5	10·7	1·8	5·8	6·3	4·4	2·4	2·0	1·4	25·4
1968	18·0	12·4	10·6	1·8	5·9	6·3	4·3	2·4	2·1	1·5	24·7
1969	18·0	12·0	10·3	1·7	6·0	6·0	4·3	2·5	2·1	1·5	23·4
1970	18·2	12·3	10·6	1·7	5·9	6·3	4·3	2·6	2·0	1·3	23·5
1971	17·5	11·6	9·9	1·7	5·9	6·0	3·9	2·6	2·0	1·3	22·3
1972	17·2	11·5	9·8	1·7	5·7	5·8	4·1	2·4	2·0	1·4	21·7
1973	16·9	11·1	9·5	1·6	5·7	5·5	4·0	2·5	1·9	1·3	21·0
1974	16·3	11·0	9·4	1·7	5·3	5·2	4·2	2·3	1·9	1·1	20·4

Source: OPCS
Registrar General's Statistical Review

[1] Rates based on related live births from 1926 to 1956.

[2] The births upon which these rates are based for successive calendar years are numbers registered up to 1938 inclusive, and numbers of occurrences from 1939.

STILL BIRTHS AND INFANT DEATHS

By Hospital Region—1963, 1966, 1971, 1972 and 1973

Table C.3

England and Wales

Hospital Region[1]	Infant Deaths						Infant Mortality Rates per 1,000 live births					Rates per 1,000 total births		
	Still births	0 days	1–6 days	1–3 weeks	1–11 months	Total under 1 year	0 days	1–6 days	1–3 weeks	1–11 months	Total under 1 year	Still births	Still births plus infant deaths under 1 week	Still births plus infant deaths under 1 year
England and Wales														
1963	14,989	6,170	4,328	1,675	5,869	18,042	7·22	5·07	1·96	6·87	21·13	17·25	29·33	38·01
1966	13,243	5,564	3,882	1,487	5,214	16,147	6·55	4·57	1·75	6·14	19·00	15·34	26·29	34·05
1971	9,899	4,680	3,070	1,363	4,607	13,720	5·98	3·92	1·74	5·88	17·52	12·48	22·25	29·78
1972	8,799	4,179	2,965	1,231	4,123	12,498	5·76	4·09	1·70	5·68	17·23	11·98	21·71	29·01
1973	7,936	3,732	2,706	1,090	3,879	11,407	5·52	4·00	1·61	5·74	16·88	11·60	21·02	28·28
Newcastle														
1963	1,114	487	303	113	389	1,292	8·64	5·38	2·01	6·90	22·92	19·38	33·13	41·86
1966	906	363	255	126	395	1,139	6·80	4·78	2·36	7·40	21·34	16·69	28·08	37·68
1971	655	295	197	102	334	928	6·00	4·01	2·07	6·79	18·87	13·14	23·02	31·77
1972	549	298	213	109	247	867	6·69	4·78	2·45	5·54	19·45	12·17	23·49	31·38
1973	496	240	170	70	249	729	5·84	4·13	1·70	6·05	17·72	11·92	21·77	29·43
Leeds														
1963	976	459	303	145	463	1,370	8·14	5·38	2·57	8·21	24·31	17·02	30·31	40·91
1966	875	392	298	104	437	1,231	7·06	5·37	1·87	8·87	22·17	15·51	27·75	37·34
1971	665	329	207	95	418	1,049	6·20	3·90	1·79	7·88	19·77	12·38	22·36	31·91
1972	668	320	204	76	332	932	6·58	4·20	1·56	6·83	19·18	13·56	24·19	32·47
1973	532	287	220	73	315	895	6·40	4·90	1·62	7·00	19·05	11·72	22·88	31·42

1963	1,506	572	399	134	645	1,750	6·93	4·83	1·62	7·81	21·19	17·91	29·43	38·71
1966	1,349	588	395	136	587	1,706	7·12	4·78	1·65	7·11	20·66	16·07	27·79	36·40
1971	956	542	292	126	500	1,460	6·98	3·76	1·62	6·44	18·80	12·16	22·77	30·73
1972	905	420	293	117	466	1,296	5·92	4·13	1·65	6·57	18·27	12·60	22·52	30·64
1973	819	340	246	107	365	1,058	5·16	3·73	1·62	5·54	16·05	12·27	21·05	28·12
East Anglian														
1963	456	158	134	45	141	478	5·88	4·99	1·67	5·25	17·78	16·68	27·36	34·17
1966	381	168	116	45	152	481	6·09	4·20	1·63	5·51	17·43	13·62	23·77	30·81
1971	312	155	98	49	119	421	5·53	3·50	1·75	4·25	15·03	11·02	19·95	25·88
1972	315	137	82	47	146	412	5·06	3·03	1·74	5·39	15·21	11·50	19·49	26·54
1973	262	119	83	40	114	356	4·50	3·14	1·51	4·31	13·46	9·81	17·37	23·13
NW Metropolitan														
1963	1,235	521	366	125	420	1,432	6·60	4·63	1·58	5·32	18·13	15·39	26·45	33·24
1966	1,041	520	311	119	400	1,350	6·65	3·98	1·52	5·12	17·28	13·15	23·64	30·20
1971	727	335	262	140	378	1,115	5·07	3·96	2·12	5·72	16·87	10·88	19·82	27·57
1972	644	284	235	95	299	913	4·63	3·83	1·55	4·87	14·87	10·38	18·75	25·10
1973	598	264	230	87	281	862	4·69	4·09	1·55	4·99	15·31	10·51	19·20	25·67
NE Metropolitan														
1963	977	401	278	118	360	1,157	6·78	4·70	2·00	6·09	19·57	16·26	27·55	35·51
1966	827	366	242	69	284	961	6·25	4·13	1·18	4·85	16·41	13·92	24·16	30·10
1971	643	334	197	96	248	875	6·31	3·72	1·81	4·68	16·53	12·00	21·91	28·33
1972	582	287	173	87	253	800	5·81	3·50	1·76	5·12	16·20	11·65	20·85	27·66
1973	524	268	163	86	250	767	5·79	3·52	1·86	5·40	16·57	11·19	20·40	27·57
SE Metropolitan														
1963	965	399	277	107	368	1,151	6·84	4·75	1·83	6·31	19·73	16·27	27·67	35·68
1966	807	334	226	83	298	941	5·82	3·94	1·45	5·19	16·38	13·86	23·47	30·01
1971	583	263	179	60	230	732	5·21	3·54	1·19	4·55	14·50	11·41	20·07	25·74
1972	461	247	187	65	224	723	5·28	4·00	1·39	4·79	15·47	9·76	18·96	25·08
1973	491	218	162	53	229	662	4·95	3·68	1·20	5·20	15·02	11·02	19·55	25·88

Source: OPCS
Registrar General's Statistical Review

[1] Deaths of infants are assigned to the region of usual residence of the parents if that is within England and Wales. Before 1972 deaths of infants whose parents were normally resident outside England and Wales were assigned to the region of occurrence. From January 1972 these deaths have been included in national totals but excluded from regional figures.

STILL BIRTHS AND INFANT DEATHS

By Hospital Region—1963, 1966, 1971, 1972 and 1973

Table C.3—continued

England and Wales

Hospital Region[1]	Still births	Infant Deaths					Infant Mortality Rates per 1,000 live births					Rates per 1,000 total births		
		0 days	1-6 days	1-3 weeks	1-11 months	Total under 1 year	0 days	1-6 days	1-3 weeks	1-11 months	Total under 1 year	Still births	Still births plus infant deaths under 1 week	Still births plus infant deaths under 1 year
SW Metropolitan														
1963	725	373	238	101	326	1,038	6·82	4·35	1·85	5·96	18·99	13·09	24·12	31·83
1966	787	370	241	76	290	977	6·51	4·24	1·34	5·10	17·18	13·65	24·25	30·60
1971	537	280	165	90	228	763	5·80	3·42	1·86	4·72	15·80	11·00	20·11	26·62
1972	487	227	181	87	218	713	5·05	4·03	1·94	4·85	15·86	10·72	19·70	26·41
1973	411	212	164	68	226	670	5·11	3·96	1·64	5·45	16·17	9·82	18·80	25·83
Wessex														
1963	529	231	149	61	197	638	7·18	4·63	1·90	6·12	19·83	16·18	27·80	35·69
1966	444	208	134	58	197	597	6·33	4·08	1·76	5·99	18·16	13·33	23·60	31·25
1971	387	171	123	49	172	515	5·44	3·91	1·56	5·47	16·39	12·16	21·41	28·35
1972	317	143	113	43	166	465	4·87	3·85	1·46	5·65	15·83	10·68	19·30	26·34
1973	348	133	104	49	122	408	4·75	3·72	1·75	4·36	14·58	12·28	20·65	26·68
Oxford														
1963	526	211	154	49	185	599	6·25	4·56	1·45	5·48	17·74	15·34	25·99	32·82
1966	465	188	150	39	174	551	5·35	4·27	1·11	4·95	15·68	13·06	22·55	28·53
1971	381	187	117	54	176	534	5·43	3·40	1·57	5·11	15·50	10·94	19·67	26·27
1972	326	141	118	44	188	491	4·30	3·60	1·34	5·74	14·98	9·85	17·67	24·68
1973	300	132	104	55	137	428	4·24	3·34	1·77	4·40	13·74	9·54	17·04	23·15

		(1)	(2)	(3)	(4)	(5)	(6)	(7)	(8)	(9)	(10)	(11)	(12)	(13)	(14)
	1963	812	533	203	97	266	847	5·73	3·73	1·94	5·22	16·61	14·14	23·46	30·52
	1966	731	292	190	99	250	742	4·63	3·77	1·96	5·26	15·62	11·61	19·92	27·05
	1971	558	220	179	93	256	725	4·51	4·33	1·68	5·74	16·26	11·13	19·87	27·21
	1972	502	201	193	75	223	644	4·06	4·04	1·73	5·21	15·04	10·97	18·99	25·85
	1973	475	174	173	74										
Birmingham	1963	1,758	655	453	200	635	1,943	7·04	4·87	2·15	6·83	20·89	18·55	30·24	39·05
	1966	1,620	644	424	193	575	1,836	6·83	4·50	2·05	6·10	19·48	16·90	28·04	36·05
	1971	1,218	514	391	148	512	1,565	5·82	4·43	1·68	5·80	17·73	13·61	23·72	31·10
	1972	1,072	511	373	162	441	1,487	6·32	4·61	2·00	5·45	18·39	13·08	23·87	31·23
	1973	953	505	335	115	479	1,434	6·74	4·47	1·54	6·39	19·14	12·56	23·63	31·46
Manchester	1963	1,569	654	460	171	703	1,988	8·11	5·70	2·12	8·71	24·64	19·08	32·62	43·25
	1966	1,399	577	443	156	566	1,742	7·21	5·54	1·95	7·08	21·78	17·19	29·73	38·60
	1971	1,115	509	308	120	496	1,433	6·77	4·10	1·60	6·60	19·06	14·62	25·33	33·40
	1972	954	493	304	111	453	1,361	7·13	4·40	1·60	6·55	19·68	13·61	24·97	33·02
	1973	808	416	280	92	427	1,215	6·57	4·42	1·45	6·74	19·18	12·59	23·44	31·53
Liverpool	1963	887	385	274	84	386	1,129	8·69	6·18	1·90	8·71	25·47	19·62	34·20	44·59
	1966	761	264	222	92	299	877	6·34	5·33	2·21	7·18	21·06	17·94	29·40	38·62
	1971	543	284	170	59	281	794	7·56	4·53	1·57	7·50	21·13	14·25	26·16	35·08
	1972	473	237	134	46	205	622	6·89	3·89	1·34	5·96	18·07	13·56	24·19	31·38
	1973	420	215	140	42	227	624	6·91	4·50	1·35	7·30	20·05	13·32	24·57	33·10
Welsh	1963	954	329	337	125	365	1,156	6·99	7·16	2·66	7·76	24·58	19·88	33·76	43·97
	1966	850	290	235	92	294	911	6·46	5·24	2·05	6·55	20·30	18·59	30·08	38·52
	1971	619	262	185	82	265	794	6·09	4·30	1·90	6·15	18·44	14·17	24·41	32·35
	1972	532	222	150	61	206	639	5·56	3·75	1·53	5·16	15·99	13·14	22·33	28·92
	1973	492	203	122	71	219	615	5·40	3·24	1·89	5·82	16·36	12·92	21·45	29·06

Source: OPCS
Registrar General's Statistical Review

[1] Deaths of infants are assigned to the region of usual residence of the parents if that is within England and Wales. Before 1972 deaths of infants whose parents were normally resident outside England and Wales were assigned to the region of occurrence. From January 1972 these deaths have been included in national totals but excluded from regional figures.

INTERNATIONAL COMPARISONS OF INFANT MORTALITY RATES—1965–1973

Table C.4

Country	1965	1966	1967	1968	1969	1970	1971	1972	1973
INFANT MORTALITY[1]									
England and Wales[5]	19·0	19·0	18·3	18·3	18·0	18·2	17·5	17·2	16·9
Australia[5]	18·5	18·8	18·3	17·8	17·9	17·9	17·3	16·7	16·5
Bulgaria	30·8	32·2	33·1	28·3	30·5	27·3	24·9	26·2	25·9
Canada	23·6	23·1	22·0	20·8	19·3	18·8	17·5	17·1	15·5
Denmark	18·7[5]	16·9[5]	15·8[5]	16·4	14·8	14·2	13·5	12·2	11·5
Finland	17·6	15·0	14·8	14·4	14·3	13·2	12·7	12·0	
France	21·9	21·7	20·7	20·4	19·6	18·2	17·1	16·0	15·5
Japan	18·5	19·3	14·9	15·3	14·2	13·1	12·4	11·7	11·3
Netherlands	14·4	14·7	13·4	13·6	13·2	12·7	12·1	11·7	11·5
New Zealand[5]	19·6	17·7	18·1	18·7	16·9	16·8	16·5	15·6	16·2
Northern Ireland[5]	25·1	25·6	23·5	24·0	24·4	22·9	22·7	20·5	20·9
Norway	16·8	14·6	14·8	13·7	13·8	12·7	12·8	11·8	11·9
Scotland[5]	23·1	23·2	21·0	20·8	21·1	19·6	19·9	18·8	19·0
Sweden	13·3	12·6	12·9	13·1	11·7	11·0	11·1	10·8	9·9
Switzerland	17·8	17·1	17·5	16·1	15·4	15·1	14·4	13·3	13·2
USA	24·7	23·7	22·4	21·8	20·9	20·0	19·1	18·5	17·7
Yugoslavia	71·8	62·1	62·1	58·6	57·3	55·5	49·5	44·4	44·0
POST NEONATAL MORTALITY[2]									
England and Wales[5]	6·0	6·1	5·8	5·9	6·0	5·9	5·9	5·7	5·7
Australia[5]	5·3	5·4	4·9	4·9	5·0	5·0	5·1	4·7	4·7
Bulgaria	17·1	18·0	18·2	13·9	16·7	14·1	12·1	12·8	12·0
Canada	7·2	7·0	6·8	6·1	5·4	5·3	5·2	5·2	4·8
Denmark	4·0[5]	3·6[5]	3·7[5]	4·5	3·1	3·2	2·8	2·5	2·8
Finland	4·0	3·1	3·0	3·1	3·1	2·8	2·7	2·3	
France	6·7	6·8	6·2	6·2	5·9	5·5	5·1	4·8	
Japan	6·8	7·3	5·0	5·5	5·2	4·5	4·2	3·9	3·9
Netherlands	3·0	3·5	2·9	3·2		3·3	3·1	2·9	3·1
New Zealand[5]	7·4	6·4	6·8	6·9	6·1	6·4	5·9	5·6	6·3
Northern Ireland[5]	7·3	8·5	7·2	8·3	8·5	7·1	6·8	6·6	3·4
Norway	4·8	4·3	3·6	3·6	3·3	3·3	3·2	2·9	6·3
Scotland[5]	7·2	8·0	7·2	7·5	7·6	6·9	6·4	6·4	2·0
Sweden	2·7	2·3	2·4	2·5	2·5	1·9	2·3	2·1	3·8
Switzerland	4·0	4·0	3·9	3·7	3·9	4·2	4·4	4·3	
USA									

MORTALITY[2]

Country									
England and Wales[5]	1·7	1·7	1·8	1·7	1·8	1·7	1·7	1·7	1·6
Australia[5]	1·5	1·4	1·5	1·4	1·2	1·3	1·4	1·1	1·2
Bulgaria	5·4	5·2	6·0	5·1	4·7	4·1	4·1	4·1	4·0
Canada	1·5	1·7	1·6	1·6	1·4	1·4	1·4	1·2	1·4
Denmark	1·5[5]	1·4[5]	1·3[5]	1·3	1·4	1·5	1·4	1·4	1·4
Finland	1·3	1·3	1·4	1·4	1·5	1·3	1·1	1·2	..
France	2·4	2·5	2·2	2·5	2·5	2·4	2·3	2·1	..
Japan	3·5	3·3	2·7	2·5	2·3	2·0	1·9	1·7	1·6
Netherlands	1·3	1·6	1·3	1·4	1·4	1·4	1·3	1·4	1·2
New Zealand[5]	1·5	1·4	1·5	1·6	1·3	1·3	1·3	1·3	..
Northern Ireland[5]	2·1	2·3	2·2	2·1	2·1	2·2	2·8	2·1	2·0
Norway	2·1	1·9	1·4	2·0	1·4	0·9	1·2	0·9	1·1
Scotland[5]	1·0	1·3	1·1	1·2	2·1	1·7	2·0	1·8	1·7
Sweden	1·3	1·4	1·4	1·4	1·1	1·0	1·0	1·1	0·9
Switzerland	1·8	1·6	1·5	1·4	1·3	1·5	1·4	1·3	1·5
USA									
Yugoslavia	12·4	10·1	9·5	9·1	8·6	7·9	6·8	6·1	5·5

PERINATAL MORTALITY[4]

Country									
England and Wales[5]	26·9	26·3	25·4	24·7	23·4	23·5	22·3	21·7	21·0
Australia[5]	23·3	23·9	22·9	21·5	21·3	21·3	19·9	22·3	22·1
Bulgaria	18·2	18·8	19·6	19·1	17·6	18·8	19·1	18·5	18·9
Canada	26·0	25·5	24·7	23·7	22·3	21·8	20·1	19·0	17·6
Denmark	23·9[5]	21·6[5]	19·5[5]	18·9	18·7	17·9	17·4	16·1	14·5
Finland	24·5	21·5	20·9	19·7	18·8	17·0	16·5	16·9	..
France	27·7	27·3	26·8	25·7	25·1	23·4	22·5	21·3	17·8
Japan	29·5	30·6	25·8	24·1	22·6	21·3	20·2	18·8	16·3
Netherlands	23·1	22·4	21·1	20·2	19·6	18·6	17·6	16·6	..
New Zealand[5]	22·3	20·8	21·5	22·1	19·4	19·6	19·3	18·7	..
Northern Ireland[5]	34·5	30·8	31·3	29·4	28·8	27·6	27·2	26·0	25·6
Norway	21·3	20·8	20·5	19·7	20·2	19·1	17·7	17·5	16·6
Scotland[5]	31·5	29·3	27·5	25·9	25·2	24·8	24·5	23·7	22·5
Sweden	19·7	18·8	18·7	18·3	16·2	16·4	15·6	14·3	14·0
Switzerland	22·8	21·5	21·8	20·9	19·3	18·1	17·0	16·2	15·4
USA	28·1	27·4	26·7	26·8	24·5	23·6	22·5	22·6	..
Yugoslavia	27·9	26·7	26·5	26·1	25·7	24·7	23·4	23·4	23·2

1 Deaths of infants under one year of age per 1,000 live births.
2 Deaths of infants aged 4 weeks and under one year per 1,000 live births.
3 Deaths of infants aged 7 days and under 28 days per 1,000 live births.
4 Still births plus deaths of infants under one week per 1,000 total births.
5 Data tabulated by year of registration rather than occurrence.

Sources: WHO Statistics Annual and Publications of the countries concerned

LIVE AND STILL BIRTHS AND NEONATAL DEATHS

By Birthweight Group—1954-1974

Table C.5

England and Wales

Notified birthweight		1954	1956	1958	1960	1962	1964	1966	1968	1970	1971	1972	1973	1974
1500gr and less	Stillbirths		3,697	3,928	3,828	3,985	3,904	3,535	3,236	2,981	2,860	2,532	2,391	2,130
	Live births	5,193	5,455	5,661	5,970	6,249	6,395	5,893	5,987	5,831	5,326	4,952	4,507	4,480
	Deaths Day 0	2,332	2,411	2,543	2,798	2,969	2,793	2,660	2,393	2,293	2,118	1,912	1,697	1,607
	Deaths Days 1–28	1,224	1,223	1,242	1,173	1,128	1,152	1,045	1,097	1,010	888	814	751	738
1501–2000gr	Stillbirths		2,273	2,326	2,259	2,279	2,185	2,110	1,801	1,580	1,501	1,346	1,251	1,109
	Live births	8,451	8,711	9,228	9,503	9,797	9,958	9,759	9,687	9,460	8,826	8,415	7,689	7,309
	Deaths Day 0	769	814	862	906	905	879	806	792	745	749	632	557	498
	Deaths Days 1–28	909	790	824	741	696	709	603	564	540	481	529	428	358
2001–2250gr	Stillbirths		961	1,039	963	1,021	942	940	805	767	678	625	628	510
	Live births	9,074	9,705	10,160	10,599	11,550	11,545	11,746	11,519	11,759	11,071	10,779	9,924	9,294
	Deaths Day 0	308	313	319	382	349	360	336	282	316	284	280	267	208
	Deaths Days 1–28	428	466	385	387	393	369	316	332	290	251	230	228	191
2251–2500gr	Stillbirths		1,374	1,372	1,377	1,251	1,171	1,109	967	843	742	658	622	500
	Live births	23,300	23,641	25,693	26,561	28,403	27,954	27,807	26,987	26,464	24,663	23,795	21,479	20,247
	Deaths Day 0	364	342	400	414	416	419	349	289	308	283	242	220	226
	Deaths Days 1–28	662	575	649	484	610	438	373	377	338	310	333	246	246
All births 2500gr and less	Stillbirths		8,305	8,665	8,427	8,536	8,202	7,694	6,809	6,171	5,781	5,161	4,892	4,249
	Live births	46,018	47,512	50,742	52,633	55,999	55,852	55,205	54,180	53,514	49,886	47,941	43,599	41,330
	Deaths Day 0	3,773	3,880	4,124	4,500	4,639	4,451	4,151	3,756	3,662	3,434	3,066	2,741	2,539
	Deaths Days 1–28	3,223	3,054	3,100	2,785	2,827	2,668	2,337	2,370	2,178	1,930	1,906	1,653	1,533
All Registered Births	Stillbirths	16,200	16,405	16,288	15,819	15,464	14,546	13,243	11,848	10,345	9,899	8,799	7,936	7,175
	Live births	673,651	700,335	740,715	785,005	836,736	875,972	849,823	819,272	784,486	783,155	725,440	675,953	639,885
	Deaths Day 0	5,098	5,144	5,551	5,920	6,212	6,230	5,564	5,184	4,971	4,680	4,179	3,732	3,328
	Deaths Days 1–28	6,848	6,635	6,419	6,271	6,444	5,876	5,369	4,941	4,690	4,433	4,196	3,796	3,739
All Registered Births minus notified low weight births	Stillbirths		8,100	7,623	7,392	6,928	6,344	5,549	5,039	4,174	4,118	3,638	3,044	2,926
	Live births	627,633	652,823	689,973	732,372	780,737	820,120	794,618	765,092	730,972	733,269	677,499	632,354	598,555
	Deaths Day 0	1,325	1,264	1,427	1,420	1,573	1,779	1,413	1,428	1,309	1,246	1,113	991	789
	Deaths Days 1–28	3,625	3,581	3,319	3,486	3,617	3,208	3,032	2,571	2,512	2,503	2,290	2,143	2,206

MORTALITY RATES PER 1,000 BIRTHS

By Birthweight Group—1954–1974

Notified birthweight		1954	1956	1958	1960	1962	1964	1966	1968	1970	1971	1972	1973	1974
1500gr and less	Stillbirths		404·0	409·6	390·7	389·4	379·1	374·9	350·9	338·3	349·4	338·3	346·6	322·2
	Day 0	449·1	442·0	449·2	468·7	475·1	436·7	451·4	399·7	393·2	397·7	386·1	376·5	358·7
	Days 1–28	427·8	401·8	398·3	369·8	343·9	319·8	323·2	305·2	285·5	276·8	267·8	267·3	236·9
1501–2000gr	Stillbirths		206·9	201·3	192·1	188·7	179·9	177·8	156·8	143·1	145·3	137·9	139·9	131·7
	Day 0	91·0	93·4	93·4	95·3	92·4	88·3	82·6	81·8	78·8	84·9	75·1	72·4	68·1
	Days 1–28	118·3	100·0	98·5	86·2	78·3	78·1	67·4	63·4	62·0	59·6	68·0	60·0	52·6
2001–2250gr	Stillbirths		90·1	92·8	83·3	81·2	75·4	74·1	65·3	61·2	57·7	54·8	59·5	52·0
	Day 0	33·9	32·3	31·4	36·0	30·2	31·2	28·6	24·5	26·9	25·7	26·0	26·9	22·4
	Days 1–28	48·8	49·6	39·1	37·9	35·1	33·0	27·7	29·5	25·3	23·3	21·9	23·6	21·0
2251–2500gr	Stillbirths		54·9	50·7	49·3	42·2	40·2	38·4	34·6	30·9	29·2	26·9	28·1	24·1
	Day 0	15·6	14·5	15·6	15·6	14·6	15·0	12·6	10·7	11·6	11·5	10·2	10·2	11·2
	Days 1–28	28·9	24·7	25·7	18·5	21·8	15·9	13·6	14·1	12·9	12·7	14·1	11·6	12·3
All births 2500gr and less	Stillbirths		148·8	145·9	138·0	132·3	128·0	122·3	111·6	103·4	103·8	97·2	100·9	93·2
	Day 0	82·0	81·7	81·3	85·5	82·8	79·7	75·2	69·3	68·4	68·8	63·9	62·9	61·4
	Days 1–28	76·3	70·0	66·5	57·9	55·0	51·9	45·8	47·0	43·7	41·5	42·5	40·5	39·5
All Registered Births minus notified low weight births	Stillbirths		12·3	10·9	10·0	8·8	7·7	6·9	6·5	5·7	5·6	5·3	4·8	4·9
	Day 0	2·1	1·9	2·1	1·9	2·0	2·2	1·8	1·9	1·8	1·7	1·6	1·6	1·3
	Days 1–28	5·8	5·5	4·8	4·8	4·6	3·9	3·8	3·4	3·4	3·4	3·4	3·4	3·7
Percentage of Stillbirths	2500gr and less		50·6	53·2	53·3	55·2	56·4	58·1	57·5	59·7	58·4	58·7	61·6	59·2
Percentage of Live births	2500gr and less	6·8	6·8	6·9	6·7	6·7	6·4	6·5	6·6	6·8	6·4	6·6	6·5	6·5
Percentage of Live and Stillbirths	2500gr and less		7·8	7·8	7·6	7·6	7·2	7·3	7·3	7·5	7·0	7·2	7·1	7·0

Source: DHSS
Welsh Office

83

LOW WEIGHT BIRTHS (less than 2,500 gr.)

By Regional Health Authority—1974

Numbers and rates per 100,000 home population by cause—1951, 1961, 1966, 1971–1974

Table C.6

England and Wales

Regional Health Authority	Stillbirths	Live births					Deaths per 1,000[1]
		Total	Born in hospital	Born at home or nursing home	As percentage of all live births	Percentage born in hospital	
England and Wales	4,249	41,330	40,204	1,126	6·5	97·3	99
Northern	275	2,622	2,576	46	6·6	98·2	108
Yorkshire	357	3,149	3,071	78	6·7	97·5	106
Trent	447	3,782	3,609	173	6·4	95·4	95
East Anglian	135	1,295	1,228	67	5·4	94·8	98
NW Thames	279	2,905	2,861	44	6·4	98·5	82
NE Thames	332	3,352	3,286	66	6·7	98·0	92
SE Thames	228	2,703	2,588	115	6·1	95·7	96
SW Thames	185	1,760	1,726	34	5·2	98·1	99
Wessex	185	2,323	2,294	29	6·8	98·8	105
Oxford	150	1,699	1,669	30	5·6	98·2	92
South Western	214	2,183	2,146	37	5·7	98·3	81
West Midlands	559	5,076	4,916	160	7·2	96·8	94
Mersey	265	2,218	2,160	58	6·8	97·4	116
North Western	361	3,822	3,687	135	7·0	96·5	114
Wales	277	2,441	2,387	54	6·7	97·8	98
England and Wales							
1973	4,892	43,599	42,036	1,563	6·5	96·4	101
1972	5,161	47,941	45,717	2,224	6·6	95·4	104
1971	5,781	49,886	46,982	2,904	6·4	94·2	108
1966	7,694	55,205	47,934	7,271	6·5	86·8	118

Source: DHSS
Welsh Office

[1] Deaths in first 28 days of life only.

DEATHS OF CHILDREN AGED UNDER ONE YEAR

Numbers and rates per 100,000 live births by cause—1951, 1961, 1966, 1971–1974

Table C.7

England and Wales

ICD Number 1951, 1961¹, 1966	ICD Number 1971–1974²	Cause	Sex	Numbers 1951	1961	1966	1971	1972	1973	1974	Rates per 100,000 live births 1951	1961	1966	1971	1972	1973	1974
		All causes	M	11,773	9,988	9,357	7,974	7,210	6,599	6,137	3,377·18	2,390·80	2,139·91	1,977·57	1,927·90	1,892·58	1,862·75
			F	8,450	7,405	6,790	5,746	5,288	4,808	4,322	2,568·97	1,881·77	1,645·82	1,512·38	1,504·59	1,469·10	1,392·28
001–138, 571,764	000–136	Infective and parasitic diseases	M	854	300	319	325	267	270	217	244·98	71·81	72·95	80·60	71·39	77·44	65·87
			F	658	272	232	238	202	179	147	200·05	69·12	56·23	62·64	57·47	54·69	47·35
571, 764	008, 009	Enteritis and other diarrhoeal diseases	M	498	202	221	193	175	148	105	142·86	48·35	50·54	47·86	46·79	42·45	31·87
			F	333	185	157	127	122	107	67	101·24	47·01	38·05	33·43	34·71	32·69	21·58
140–205	140–209	Malignant neoplasms	M	32	37	22	20	25	20	17	9·18	8·86	5·03	4·96	6·68	5·74	5·16
			F	24	16	25	21	19	14	14	7·30	4·07	6·06	5·53	5·41	4·28	4·51
330–398	320–389	Diseases of the nervous system and sense organs	M	227	176	181	145	137	142	96	65·12	42·13	41·39	35·96	36·63	40·73	29·14
			F	152	129	156	114	98	102	76	46·21	32·78	37·81	30·01	27·88	31·17	24·48
470–527, 241,763	460–519	Diseases of the respiratory system	M	2,414	1,603	1,721	1,400	1,145	964	865	692·48	383·71	393·59	347·20	306·16	276·47	262·55
			F	1,793	1,176	1,186	1,028	760	656	539	545·11	298·85	287·47	270·57	216·24	200·44	173·63
470–475, 480–483, 500	470–474, 460–466	Acute respiratory infections and influenza	M	319	184	219	439	380	286	284	91·51	44·04	50·08	108·87	101·61	82·02	86·20
			F	219	125	148	331	233	204	164	66·58	31·77	35·87	87·12	66·30	62·33	32·83
490–493, 763	480–486	Pneumonia	M	1,979	1,331	1,368	821	637	565	488	567·69	318·60	312·86	203·61	170·33	162·04	148·12
			F	1,490	979	934	600	457	385	327	452·99	248·78	226·39	157·92	130·03	117·64	105·34
750–759	740–759	Congenital anomalies	M	1,536	1,846	1,707	1,594	1,405	1,305	1,284	440·61	441·87	390·38	395·31	375·69	374·27	389·73
			F	1,328	1,758	1,526	1,356	1,352	1,247	1,226	403·74	446·75	369·88	356·91	384·68	381·03	394·94
..	760–779	Certain causes of perinatal morbidity and mortality³	M	..	..	..	3,731	3,376	3,069	2,830	..	..	..	925·29	902·72	880·18	858·98
			F	..	..	..	2,428	2,255	2,015	1,777	..	..	..	639·06	641·61	615·69	572·44
E800–E962	E800–E949, E980–E989⁴	Accidents	M	435	285	355	234	186	187	150	124·78	68·22	81·19	58·03	49·74	53·63	45·53
			F	310	190	255	179	168	112	106	94·25	48·28	61·81	47·11	47·80	34·22	34·15
		All other causes	M	6,275	5,741	5,052	525	669	642	678	1,800·04	1,374·21	1,155·37	130·20	178·89	184·12	205·79
			F	4,185	3,864	3,410	382	434	483	437	1,272·33	981·92	826·54	100·54	123·49	147·58	140·77

¹ International Classification of Diseases 6th and 7th Revisions.
² International Classification of Diseases 8th Revision.
³ Comparable figures are not available for 1951, 1961 and 1966. For those years deaths are included in the numbers for "all other causes".
⁴ Deaths undetermined whether accidentally or purposely inflicted. Numbers are small: (1972: Male = 8, Female = 7). Included with accidents prior to 1968.

Source: OPCS
Registrar General's Statistical Review

DEATHS OF CHILDREN AGED 1-4 YEARS

Numbers and rates per 100,000 home population by cause—1951, 1961, 1966, 1971–1974

Table C.8 — England and Wales

ICD Number 1951, 1961,[1] 1966	ICD Number 1971–1974[2]	Cause		Numbers 1951	1961	1966	1971	1972	1973	1974	Rates per 100,000 home population 1951	1961	1966	1971	1972	1973	1974
		All causes	M	2,257	1,536	1,563	1,228	1,235	1,203	1,095	144·22	104·10	92·20	76·57	78·01	77·03	72·42
			F	1,876	1,126	1,220	976	1,073	896	827	125·74	80·56	75·33	64·10	71·33	60·50	57·84
001–138, 571	000–136	Infective and parasitic diseases	M	596	206	147	63	119	97	126	38·08	13·96	8·67	3·93	7·52	6·21	8·33
			F	532	122	124	105	93	87	82	35·66	8·73	7·66	6·90	6·18	5·87	5·73
571	008, 009	Enteritis and other diarrhoeal diseases	M	63	66	65	26	67	33	36	4·03	4·47	3·83	1·62	4·23	2·11	2·38
			F	45	26	59	47	46	42	24	3·02	1·86	3·64	3·09	3·06	2·84	1·68
140–205	140–209	Malignant neoplasms	M	175	184	184	134	143	133	117	11·18	12·47	10·85	8·36	9·03	8·52	7·74
			F	162	126	140	102	121	90	100	10·86	9·01	8·64	6·70	8·04	6·08	6·99
330–398	320–389	Diseases of the nervous system and sense organs	M	130	96	115	75	96	87	79	8·31	6·51	6·78	4·68	6·06	5·57	5·22
			F	114	73	76	55	94	70	65	7·64	5·22	4·69	3·61	6·25	4·73	4·55
470–527, 241,763	460–519	Diseases of the respiratory system	M	441	369	299	212	223	229	174	28·18	25·01	17·64	13·22	14·09	14·66	11·51
			F	423	263	282	197	205	171	136	28·35	[18·82	17·41	12·94	13·63	11·55	9·51
470–475, 480–483, 500	470–474, 460–466	Acute respiratory infections and influenza	M	105	86	67	59	69	54	44	6·71	5·83	3·95	3·68	4·36	3·46	2·91
			F	99	64	58	47	54	38	27	6·64	4·58	3·58	3·09	3·59	2·57	1·89
490–493, 763	480–486	Pneumonia	M	274	226	190	113	116	128	90	17·51	15·32	11·21	7·05	7·33	8·20	5·95
			F	280	162	192	108	110	110	82	18·77	11·59	11·85	7·09	7·31	7·43	5·73
750–759	740–759	Congenital anomalies	M	166	185	202	209	183	211	203	10·61	12·54	11·92	13·03	11·56	13·51	13·43
			F	138	184	170	186	197	179	166	9·25	13·16	10·50	12·22	13·10	12·09	11·61
E800–E949	E800–E949, E980–E989[3]	Accidents	M	472	365	449	399	337	318	263	30·16	24·74	26·48	24·88	21·29	20·36	17·39
			F	311	240	291	218	226	190	184	20·84	17·17	17·97	14·32	15·02	12·83	12·87
		All other causes	M	277	131	167	136	134	128	133	17·70	8·88	9·85	8·48	8·46	8·20	8·80
			F	196	118	137	113	137	109	94	13·14	8·44	8·46	7·42	9·11	7·36	6·57

[1] International Classification of Diseases 6th and 7th Revisions.
[2] International Classification of Diseases 8th Revision.
[3] Deaths undetermined whether accidentally or purposely inflicted. Included with accidents prior to 1968.

Source: OPCS
Registrar General's Statistical Review

DEATHS OF CHILDREN AGED 5-9 YEARS

Numbers and rates per 100,000 home population by cause—1951, 1961, 1966, 1971-1974

Table C.9   England and Wales

ICD Number 1951, 1961¹, 1966	ICD Number 1971-1974²	Cause	Sex	Numbers 1951	1961	1966	1971	1972	1973	1974	Rates per 100,000 home population 1951	1961	1966	1971	1972	1973	1974
		All causes	M	1,072	803	823	916	847	817	720	65·29	48·01	43·87	44·06	40·65	39·48	35·26
			F	699	517	518	568	579	510	505	44·58	32·47	29·29	28·77	29·22	25·93	26·00
000-136	001-138, 571	Infective and parasitic diseases	M	159	53	34	30	18	25	24	9·68	3·17	1·81	1·44	0·86	1·21	1·18
			F	138	46	28	21	23	26	20	8·80	2·89	1·58	1·06	1·16	1·32	1·03
008, 009	571	Enteritis and other diarrhoeal diseases	M	8	4	5	5	3	5	5	0·49	0·24	0·27	0·24	0·14	0·24	0·24
			F	6	6	3	4	1	3	5	0·38	0·38	0·17	0·20	0·05	0·15	0·26
140-209	140-205	Malignant neoplasms	M	126	120	137	157	160	147	138	7·67	7·18	7·30	7·55	7·68	7·10	6·76
			F	85	107	96	130	111	95	88	5·42	6·72	5·41	6·59	5·60	4·83	4·53
320-389	330-398	Diseases of the nervous system and sense organs	M	58	57	51	46	56	48	43	3·53	3·41	2·72	2·21	2·69	2·32	2·11
			F	54	44	33	34	45	38	37	3·44	2·76	1·86	1·72	2·27	1·93	1·90
460-519	470-527, 241, 763	Diseases of the respiratory system	M	90	74	74	71	75	50	47	5·48	4·42	3·94	3·42	3·60	2·42	2·30
			F	94	62	72	57	55	39	51	5·99	3·89	4·07	2·89	2·78	1·98	2·63
470-474, 460-466	470-475, 480-483, 500, 763	Acute respiratory infections and influenza	M	17	19	16	6	19	6	5	1·04	1·14	0·85	0·29	0·91	0·29	0·24
			F	19	11	19	10	14	8	7	1·21	0·69	1·07	0·51	0·71	0·41	0·36
480-486	490-493, 763	Pneumonia	M	47	39	38	46	38	32	34	2·86	2·33	2·03	2·21	1·82	1·55	1·67
			F	39	41	40	38	31	22	39	2·49	2·58	2·26	1·93	1·56	1·12	2·01
740-759	750-759	Congenital anomalies	M	57	72	65	94	61	85	76	3·47	4·31	3·46	4·52	2·93	4·11	3·72
			F	38	64	58	76	85	85	84	2·42	4·02	3·27	3·85	4·29	4·32	4·32
E800-E949, E980-E989³	E800-E962	Accidents	M	420	326	359	391	388	355	291	25·58	19·49	19·13	18·81	18·62	17·15	14·25
			F	145	111	140	161	168	147	151	9·25	6·97	7·89	8·16	8·48	7·47	7·77
		All other causes	M	162	101	103	127	89	107	101	9·87	6·04	5·49	6·11	4·27	5·17	4·95
			F	145	83	91	89	92	80	74	9·25	5·21	5·13	4·51	4·64	4·07	3·81

¹ International Classification of Diseases 6th and 7th Revisions.
² International Classification of Diseases 8th Revision.
³ Deaths undetermined whether accidentally or purposely inflicted. Included with accidents prior to 1968.

Source: OPCS.
Registrar General's Statistical Review

DEATHS OF CHILDREN AGED 10–14 YEARS

Numbers and rates per 100,000 home population by cause—1951, 1961, 1966, 1971–1974

Table C.10 England and Wales

ICD Number 1951, 1961¹, 1966	ICD Number 1971–1974²	Cause	M/F	Numbers 1951	1961	1966	1971	1972	1973	1974	Rates per 100,000 home population 1951	1961	1966	1971	1972	1973	1974
		All causes	M	812	745	706	690	693	677	649	57·10	39·48	44·98	36·82	36·07	34·40	32·20
			F	516	441	398	419	367	393	442	37·47	24·51	25·06	23·66	20·17	21·06	23·14
001–138, 571	000–136	Infective and parasitic diseases	M	87	30	21	10	8	14	14	6·12	1·59	1·25	0·53	0·42	0·71	0·69
			F	104	22	18	13	6	20	14	7·55	1·22	1·13	0·73	0·33	1·07	0·73
571	008, 009	Enteritis and other diarrhoeal diseases	M	1	4	1	2	2	—	1	0·07	0·21	0·06	0·11	0·10	—	0·05
			F	—	1	4	2	—	—	2	0·07	0·06	0·25	0·11	—	—	0·10
140–205	140–209	Malignant neoplasms	M	100	119	109	113	129	128	103	7·03	6·31	6·48	6·03	6·71	6·50	5·11
			F	58	98	74	85	53	78	81	4·21	5·45	4·66	4·80	2·91	4·18	4·24
330–398	320–389	Diseases of the nervous system and sense organs	M	72	57	43	43	50	51	54	5·06	3·02	2·56	2·29	2·60	2·59	2·68
			F	40	39	30	22	24	23	30	2·90	2·17	1·89	1·24	1·32	1·23	1·57
470–527, 241, 763	460–519	Diseases of the respiratory system	M	55	65	101	48	50	50	55	3·87	3·44	6·01	2·56	2·60	2·54	2·73
			F	49	69	71	47	48	45	38	3·56	3·84	4·47	2·65	2·64	2·41	1·99
470–475, 480–483, 500	470–474, 460–466	Acute respiratory infections and influenza	M	13	13	12	7	8	5	10	0·91	0·69	0·71	0·37	0·42	0·25	0·50
			F	15	20	9	4	11	6	7	1·09	1·11	0·57	0·23	0·60	0·32	0·37
490–493, 763	480–486	Pneumonia	M	23	32	38	23	23	23	29	1·62	1·70	2·26	1·23	1·20	1·17	1·44
			F	22	28	21	33	26	30	20	1·60	1·56	1·32	1·86	1·43	1·61	1·05
750–759	740–759	Congenital anomalies	M	47	77	39	66	56	52	49	3·31	4·08	2·32	3·52	2·91	2·64	2·43
			F	28	39	34	46	36	31	52	2·03	2·17	2·14	2·60	1·98	1·66	2·72
E800–E962	E800–E949, E980–E989³	Accidents	M	262	294	307	316	288	257	253	18·42	15·58	18·26	16·86	14·99	13·06	12·55
			F	61	70	102	123	97	102	115	4·43	3·89	6·42	6·94	5·33	5·47	6·02
		All other causes	M	189	103	86	94	112	125	121	13·29	5·46	5·11	5·02	5·83	6·35	6·00
			F	176	104	69	83	103	94	112	12·78	5·78	4·34	4·69	5·66	5·04	5·86

¹ International Classification of Diseases 6th and 7th Revisions.
² International Classification of Diseases 8th Revision.
³ Deaths undetermined whether accidentally or purposely inflicted. Included with accidents prior to 1968.

Source: OPCS
Registrar General's Statistical Review

DEATHS OF CHILDREN AGED 15–19 YEARS

By sex and type of birth: rates per 10,000 births—1970–1974

Table C.11

England and Wales

ICD Number 1951, 1961¹, 1966	ICD Number 1971–1974²	Cause	Sex	Numbers 1951	1961	1966	1971	1972	1973	1974	Rates per 100,000 home population 1951	1961	1966	1971	1972	1973	1974
		All causes	M	1,181	1,517	2,001	1,538	1,482	1,510	1,582	88·60	92·10	107·51	90·38	85·65	86·08	88·83
			F	880	620	737	631	658	681	630	64·23	38·68	40·73	38·94	40·04	40·81	37·07
001–138, 571	000–136	Infective and parasitic diseases	M	165	27	23	24	17	33	27	12·38	1·64	1·24	1·41	0·98	1·88	1·52
			F	264	19	18	17	19	19	16	19·27	1·18	0·99	1·05	1·16	1·14	0·94
571	008, 009	Enteritis and other diarrhoeal diseases	M	2	1	1	—	1	2	2	0·15	0·06	0·05	—	0·06	0·11	0·11
			F	1	1	1	—	2	5	1	0·07	0·06	0·06	—	0·12	0·30	0·06
140–205	140–209	Malignant neoplasms	M	99	149	183	121	126	137	141	7·43	9·05	9·83	7·11	7·28	7·81	7·92
			F	64	75	122	90	88	106	90	4·67	4·68	6·74	5·55	5·35	6·35	5·30
330–398	320–389	Diseases of the nervous system and sense organs	M	78	80	81	89	75	75	89	5·85	4·86	4·35	5·23	4·33	4·28	5·00
			F	59	39	53	30	34	43	39	4·31	2·43	2·93	1·85	2·07	2·58	2·29
470–527, 241, 763	460–519	Diseases of the respiratory system	M	94	83	136	84	89	80	92	7·05	5·04	7·31	4·94	5·14	4·56	5·17
			F	79	66	104	61	58	54	46	5·77	4·12	5·75	3·76	3·53	3·24	2·71
470–475, 480–483, 500, 763	470–474, 460–466	Acute respiratory infections and influenza	M	24	22	14	7	16	10	13	1·80	1·34	0·75	0·41	0·92	0·57	0·73
			F	18	19	13	6	10	9	2	1·31	1·19	0·72	0·37	0·61	0·54	0·12
490–493, 763	480–486	Pneumonia	M	42	36	58	42	45	41	57	3·15	2·19	3·12	2·47	2·60	2·34	3·20
			F	27	27	33	29	29	33	27	1·97	1·68	1·82	1·79	1·76	1·98	1·59
750–759	740–759	Congenital anomalies	M	38	36	50	48	39	37	50	2·85	2·19	2·69	2·82	2·25	2·11	2·81
			F	31	41	22	30	25	24	29	2·26	2·56	1·22	1·85	1·52	1·44	1·71
E800–E962	E800–E949, E980–E989³	Accidents	M	443	910	1,232	940	938	921	980	33·23	55·25	66·19	55·24	54·21	52·50	55·03
			F	102	195	220	255	271	262	242	7·45	12·17	12·16	15·73	16·49	15·70	14·24
		All other causes	M	264	232	296	232	198	227	203	19·80	14·08	15·90	13·63	11·44	12·94	11·40
			F	281	185	198	148	163	173	168	20·51	11·54	10·94	9·13	9·92	10·37	9·89

¹ International Classification of Diseases 6th and 7th Revisions.
² International Classification of Diseases 8th Revision.
³ Deaths undetermined whether accidentally or purposely inflicted. Included with accidents prior to 1968.

Source: OPCS.
Registrar General's Statistical Review

89

NUMBER OF CHILD DEATHS AND RATES PER 100,000 PER YEAR

By age and social class—1959–1963

Table C.12   England and Wales

Age		Social Class				
		I	II	III	IV	V
All Causes						
*1–4	Numbers ...	436	1,329	6,147	2,324	1,521
	Rates ...	69·0	73·4	88·7	93·3	154·0
*5–9	Numbers ...	209	818	3,243	1,234	744
	Rates ...	32·8	35·1	41·1	41·4	66·6
*10–14	Numbers ...	173	823	2,771	1,091	555
	Rates ...	29·6	28·8	31·3	30·3	41·4
Congenital Abnormalities (ICD 750–759)						
*1–4	Numbers ...	68	197	920	274	174
	Rates ...	10·77	10·89	13·28	11·00	17·62
5–9	Numbers ...	24	91	327	117	64
	Rates ...	3·76	3·90	4·14	3·92	5·73
10–14	Numbers ...	17	83	257	94	36
	Rates ...	2·91	2·91	2·91	2·61	2·68
Respiratory Diseases (ICD 470–527)						
*1–4	Numbers ...	102	315	1,420	627	360
	Rates ...	16·15	17·41	20·49	21·15	34·46
5–9	Numbers ...	36	89	369	132	62
	Rates ...	5·65	3·81	4·67	4·43	5·55
10–14	Numbers ...	11	71	266	91	46
	Rates ...	1·88	2·49	3·01	2·52	3·43
Accidents, Poisonings and Violence (ICD E800–E999)						
*1–4	Numbers ...	60	231	1,169	598	443
	Rates ...	9·50	12·77	16·87	24·00	44·86
*5–9	Numbers ...	40	227	1,002	480	323
	Rates ...	6·28	9·73	12·68	16·10	28·90
*10–14	Numbers ...	43	231	858	405	208
	Rates ...	7·36	8·09	9·70	11·23	15·50

Source: OPCS

* Social Class differences are significant at 0·1 % level, otherwise differences are not significant.

Section D

MORBIDITY

Morbidity or illness is much harder to define than death and consequently more difficult to identify and measure. Illness is not always reported to general practitioners and, when it is, a precise description or diagnosis may not be recorded. Moreover, general practitioners will differ in the extent to which they encourage patients to consult them and the extent to which they themselves refer patients to hospital consultants with the result that, although morbidity treated in hospitals is well recorded, for in-patients at any rate, it may not be a valid reflection of the extent of morbidity in the population. The various statistics in this section, derived from a variety of sources, are all, therefore, in many ways inadequate for measuring the prevalence and incidence of child morbidity and describing its characteristics.

The General Household Survey obtains some information on the prevalence of chronic disability in childhood and the incidence of acute illness. The 1973 survey showed that about 5% of children aged 0–4 were reported to be suffering from long standing illness; in between 1% and 2% of children this illness limited their activity in some way. For children aged 5–14 the rates were somewhat higher, 9% of boys and 7% of girls were reported as chronically sick, of which 4% of boys and 3% of girls were reported as limited in some way by the condition. However, the extent of limitation will vary between conditions and between groups of the population, depending on their relative perception of the illness and its consequences.

Acute illness in the last fortnight before the survey interview was reported for about 7% of children aged 0–14, there being no marked difference between boys and girls or between older and younger children. These illnesses led on average to about 10 restricted days per child per year. Against this background we can examine the available medical statistics on child illness.

Firstly, Tables D.1–3 provide information derived from the notifications of birth to Area Medical Officers about the number of newly-born children with congenital abnormalities. Notification is not compulsory and relates only to those abnormalities observable at birth. Reporting may not be complete and may vary between regions. Moreover, early diagnosis may be inaccurate. Although the figures reported for some malformations are probably understated there is known to be over-reporting of others which are difficult to diagnose such as talipes or congenital dislocation of the hip. The increases shown in Tables D.1 and 3 are likely to be due to improvements in data collection rather than to real increases in the incidence of malformation. Table D.2 shows the change in number of congenital abnormalities reported by type of abnormality while D.3 shows the extent of regional variation. There is considerable fluctuation from year to year, part of which at least is probably due to reporting vagaries.

Tables D.4 and 5 have been derived from "Statistics of Infectious Diseases 1974" published by the Office of Population Censuses and Surveys in Series MB2 No 1 and previous statistical reviews of the Registrar General. The first table, D.4, shows the recent historical trend in the notifications of diseases affecting children aged 0–14. D.5 provides greater detail by age and sex for

1974. These tables point to a substantial decline in the notification of infective jaundice (made notifiable in June 1968) and of measles, associated with the introduction of measles vaccine, and to less spectacular but real declines in the past 10 years in dysentery, tuberculosis, whooping cough and scarlet fever. On the other hand, notifications of acute meningitis have increased recently due to the epidemic of meningococcal infection. Statistics based on notification of infectious diseases are known to underestimate the incidence of some of these diseases, although in others there is little objective evidence of the extent of under-notification. However, this does not seriously hinder their use in the monitoring of national trends and disease patterns and epidemics at local level.

Tables D.6 and 7 deal with dental disease and have been derived from the Child Dental Health Survey of England and Wales carried out in 1973.

Table D.6 shows the percentage of children at each age whose teeth have active decay requiring treatment and who need some dental attention. It shows that the proportion of children with no known tooth decay declines very rapidly from 29% at age 5 to 3% at age 15 and that at all ages from 5 to 14 the proportion with active decay is over 60%, being as high as 78% at age 8. Moreover, Table D.7 shows that the average number of teeth with known decay experience increases with the age of the child from 3·4 at age 5 to 8·4 at age 15 and also that the proportion of total decay treated by conservation rather than extraction rises from 21% at age 5 to 71% at age 15. There are marked regional differences in the extent to which children have some permanent teeth extracted. The proportion is much higher in Wales (22% at age 10 and 50% at age 14) and much lower in London and the South East (9% at age 10 and 18% at age 14) than in the North and Midlands (16% at age 10 and 37% at age 14).

Tables D.8–13 are all derived from the Hospital In-patient Enquiry, a regular annual analysis of the characteristics of 10% of patients discharged from non-psychiatric hospitals. This is the main source of statistics about the types of illness treated in hospitals (ie. for in-patients; there is no corresponding national analysis for patients treated only in out-patient or casualty departments).

D.8 provides some data on the morbidity of babies discharged from special care baby units and gives an indication of the extent to which children under one year of age are treated in such units. This proportion is high, nearly 100% for diseases which are causes of perinatal morbidity but understandably perhaps is lower for other causes, 23·5%, for example, for congenital anomalies. Causes of perinatal morbidity account for nearly three-quarters of the cases treated in special care baby units.

D.9 provides similar information on the pattern of morbidity treated in paediatric departments and on the extent to which paediatric departments care for children aged 0–14 in different diagnostic categories. Taking all causes together, it will be seen that paediatric departments deal with 27% of discharges and deaths of children aged 0–14 but there is marked variation by cause, being as high as 88% for chemical poisoning (A149) and as low as 14% for congenital anomalies (A126–130) and diseases of the digestive system (A97–104).

Tables D.10, 11 and 12 provide a detailed comprehensive set of tables on hospital activity for children aged 0–19, setting out respectively discharge rates, average daily bed rates and mean duration of stay for different age/sex groups by selected diagnostic groups. An indication is provided of the extent of change between 1968 and 1973. Overall discharges and deaths have increased only slightly since 1968 but the falling birth rate has reduced the numbers under one year by comparison with earlier years. Causes for which there have been noticeable increases include diseases of the ear, causes of perinatal morbidity, congenital anomalies, intracranial injury and adverse effects of chemical substances. By contrast, discharge rates have fallen for respiratory diseases and hernia. Mean length of stay has fallen for all disease categories with the result that average daily bed rates per million children have also fallen except for certain causes of perinatal morbidity, symptoms and ill-defined conditions, intracranial injury (girls) and adverse effects of chemical substances.

The pattern of morbidity by age can be seen by reading across Tables D.10 and 11. Under one year of age the causes of perinatal morbidity predominate, with congenital anomalies, diseases of the respiratory system and infective and parasitic diseases being the other important groups. As age increases diseases of the respiratory system take over as the main cause of admission, followed by accidents and injuries, for children aged 1–4 and 5–9. For the 10–12 and 13–14 age groups, respiratory diseases seem slightly less important than diseases of the digestive system as a cause of admission, while accidents and injuries have become the most important cause. Admission rates are at their lowest for this age group but they increase sharply, particularly for girls of 15–19. The main reason, of course, is childbirth and complications of childbirth, not singled out for special mention in the table. Male discharge rates are higher too for the 15–19 group and again it is noticeable that there is a marked increase in accidents and injuries (A138–150) in this age group, probably as a result of road accidents.

Table D.13 provides some regional data on discharge rates for broad diagnostic categories. It will be seen that there are marked regional variations for both males and females for each cause.

There has been a steep increase in the number of known cases of sexually-transmitted diseases among adolescents, especially among girls. Table D.14 provides a comparison over nine years.

Table D.15 provides information on the child morbidity treated in general practice and revealed by the National Morbidity Survey of 1970–71. In this survey some 50 volunteer general practices provided information on patient contacts to the OPCS for a whole year. It will be seen that nearly 90% of children aged 0–4 and over 60% of children aged 5–14 were seen by their general practitioners during the year. There seems to have been a decrease since the previous study in 1955–56 when it was found that just under 75% of children under 15 consulted in the course of the year. In the current study over half the children aged 0–4 and nearly one-third aged 5–14 were seen in connection with a respiratory disease. Skin diseases and acute otitis media were also important reasons for consulting a gp but the category of symptoms and ill-defined conditions led to consultations for a quarter of the 0–4s and 14% of the 5–14s and this illustrates the fact that a precise diagnosis of the cause of morbidity is often not possible either in general practice or in hospital.

Tables D.16 and 17 give the number of children and young people in receipt of an attendance allowance. This allowance is a tax-free cash benefit for people who are severely disabled physically or mentally and require a lot of attention or supervision from another person. It is payable to adults and for children of at least two years of age and is payable in addition to most other benefits.

There are two rates. To qualify for the higher allowance, a person must be so severely disabled, physically or mentally, that for six months or more he has required by day frequent attention or continual supervision to avoid substantial danger and at night prolonged or repeated attention or again continual supervision to avoid substantial danger. To qualify for the lower allowance a person must satisfy one of the day conditions or one of the night conditions. A child under the age of 16 must satisfy the additional requirement that the attention or supervision needed is substantially in excess of that normally required by a child of the same age and sex.

The allowance at what is now called the higher rate was introduced with effect from 6 December 1971. The lower rate was introduced in stages by age groups during 1973.

Table D.16 shows the regional distribution of the attendance allowance payroll in respect of children aged 2–19; here the regional figures are for the standard statistical regions and not for health or hospital regions. Table D.17 analyses the child recipients of attendance allowance by their main cause of helplessness. At mid-1974, 15½ thousand children had qualified for benefit at the higher rate and 7,000 at the lower rate. Generally prevalence was highest, for higher rate awards, for children aged 5–9, falling away as age increased. For lower rate awards the prevalence was greatest for ages 2–4, falling away again as age rose except for ages 15–19 where there was a slight rise. The most important causes of helplessness were congenital anomalies, which accounted for more than a third of all awards, and mental disorders which accounted for only slightly less.

NOTIFIED CONGENITAL MALFORMATIONS—1964–1974

Number of babies with one or more malformation notified each year

Table D.1   England and Wales

Year	Total	Live born	Stillborn	Not stated
1964	14,631	12,335	2,225	71
1965	13,913	11,687	2,224	2
1966	13,665	11,578	2,086	1
1967	14,062	12,029	2,033	—
1968	13,954	12,071	1,883	—
1969	13,959	12,106	1,853	—
1970	14,019	12,285	1,734	—
1971	14,407	12,567	1,840	—
1972	14,412	12,782	1,629	1
1973	13,353	11,920	1,431	2
1974[1]	12,730	10,393	2,304	33

[1] Provisional.   Source: OPCS

CONGENITAL MALFORMATIONS
NUMBER OF BABIES BORN WITH EACH TYPE OF MALFORMATION

By sex and type of birth: rates per 10,000—births 1970–1974

Table D.2

England and Wales

| Site | Number of malformations | | | | | Liveborn malformation rate per 10,000 live births | | All babies[2] malformation rate per 10,000 live and still births | Index of total rate (1969=100) |
| | Live | | Still | | Total[1] | Male | Female | | |
	Male	Female	Male	Female					
All babies									
1970	6,748	5,498	645	1,067	14,019	167·3	144·3	176·4	102
1971	6,977	5,557	679	1,133	14,407	173·0	146·3	181·7	105
1972	7,049	5,679	582	1,011	14,412	188·5	161·6	196·3	114
1973	6,658	5,222	556	850	13,353	190·9	159·6	195·3	113
1974[3]	5,772	4,543	964	1,268	12,730	175·2	146·3	196·7	114
Central nervous system									
1970	821	962	467	918	3,183	20·4	25·2	40·0	98
1971	862	1,001	504	992	3,378	21·4	26·3	42·6	104
1972	805	946	453	905	3,129	21·5	26·9	42·6	104
1973	634	780	414	712	2,553	18·2	23·8	37·3	91
1974[3]	439	522	523	928	2,452	13·3	16·8	37·9	93
Eye									
1970	52	53	4	8	118	1·3	1·4	1·5	100
1971	56	42	6	3	107	1·4	1·1	1·3	87
1972	56	73	3	5	138	1·5	2·1	1·9	127
1973	44	44	4	7	99	1·3	1·3	1·4	93
1974[3]	36	46	13	15	111	1·1	1·5	1·7	112
Ear									
1970	185	147	5	9	346	4·6	3·9	4·4	102
1971	205	179	4	4	393	5·1	4·7	5·0	116
1972	224	177	9	2	413	6·0	5·0	5·6	130
1973	218	163	5	5	393	6·3	5·0	5·7	133
1974[3]	151	138	25	18	338	4·6	4·4	5·2	121

	c1	c2	c3	c4	c5	c6	c7	c8	c9
1970	618	429	28	24	1,103	15·3	11·3	13·3	99
1971	603	386	28	44	1,063	15·0	10·2	13·4	96
1972	543	384	32	35	997	14·5	10·9	13·6	97
1973	528	396	31	30	985	15·1	12·1	14·4	103
1974³	495	349	68	52	974	15·0	11·2	15·1	108
Intestines									
1970	322	205	22	13	569	8·0	5·4	7·2	118
1971	293	206	7	19	532	7·3	5·4	6·7	110
1972	246	206	21	10	497	6·6	5·9	6·8	111
1973	260	155	12	18	448	7·5	4·7	6·6	108
1974³	183	124	62	34	421	5·6	4·0	6·5	107
Cardio-vascular system									
1970	392	321	13	11	740	9·7	8·4	9·3	119
1971	382	314	11	5	714	9·5	8·3	9·0	115
1972	399	382	8	10	803	10·7	10·9	10·9	140
1973	370	335	9	7	725	10·6	10·2	10·6	136
1974³	256	238	81	66	652	7·8	7·7	10·1	129
External genitals									
1970	856	65	15	2	942	21·2	1·7	11·9	97
1971	1,031	84	11	5	1,136	25·6	2·2	14·3	116
1972	1,093	66	18	—	1,182	29·2	1·9	16·1	131
1973	1,029	77	17	—	1,125	29·5	2·4	16·5	134
1974³	949	51	35	6	1,056	28·8	1·6	16·3	133
Limbs									
1970	2,589	2,515	76	91	5,285	64·2	66·0	66·5	97
1971	2,524	2,509	70	88	5,206	62·6	66·0	65·6	96
1972	2,459	2,452	94	88	5,116	65·8	69·8	69·7	102
1973	2,227	2,208	84	71	4,611	63·9	67·5	67·4	99
1974³	1,989	1,935	200	157	4,338	60·4	62·3	67·0	98
Chromosomes									
1970	271	321	16	16	627	6·7	8·4	7·9	111
1971	278	323	13	17	632	6·9	8·5	8·0	113
1972	255	332	13	13	615	6·8	9·4	8·4	118
1973	269	278	8	16	571	7·7	8·5	8·3	117
1974³	192	203	43	32	474	5·8	6·5	7·3	103

¹Includes cases where the sex or type of birth was either indeterminate or not stated.
²Live and stillborn babies with one or more malformations.
³1974 figures are provisional.

Source: OPCS

97

CONGENITAL MALFORMATIONS IN 1974[1]

Rates[2] and certain indices for selected sites by Standard Region—1971-1974

Table D.3   England and Wales

Standard Region	Central Nervous System Rate	Eye Rate	Ear Rate	Cleft lip and/or Cleft palate Rate	Intestines Rate	Cardio-vascular system Rate	External genitals Rate	Limbs Rate	Chromosomes Rate	All babies[3] Numbers	All babies[3] Rates	Indices of rates based on 1969=100 1971	1972	1973	1974[1]
North	39·9	2·2	6·2	11·9	8·7	18·3	18·8	69·6	5·2	812	201·2	116	120	116	124
Yorkshire and Humberside ...	47·0	0·8	4·8	15·1	7·8	9·5	18·3	77·5	6·7	1,416	219·8	121	114	110	125
North West	38·9	1·0	6·1	15·5	5·3	7·4	13·3	61·6	6·1	1,678	190·6	101	115	114	112
East Midlands ...	48·8	2·2	5·1	18·6	7·1	13·8	24·9	74·4	9·3	1,276	251·9	98	117	136	139
West Midlands ...	37·9	2·5	2·7	14·1	6·9	12·7	12·5	67·5	8·5	1,331	187·5	92	112	111	110
East Anglia	24·5	2·1	5·0	15·8	6·2	5·8	15·0	57·8	9·6	392	163·1	128	123	105	98
South East	31·2	1·7	5·8	15·3	6·1	9·4	17·3	67·2	7·7	4,184	191·2	106	114	113	110
South West	39·8	1·9	6·7	13·1	7·2	9·1	13·1	69·4	7·2	1,054	200·5	103	107	111	113
Wales	48·9	1·6	2·7	15·6	4·9	6·6	12·8	50·8	5·2	586	160·0	93	105	97	94
England and Wales Total	37·9	1·7	5·2	15·1	6·5	10·1	16·3	67·1	7·3	12,730	196·7	105	114	113	114
Numbers	2,452	111	338	974	421	652	1,056	4,338	474	.	.	.	.	.	.

[1] 1974 figures are provisional.
[2] Rates per 10,000 total live and still births.
[3] Live and stillborn babies with one or more congenital malformations.

Source: OPCS

98

INFECTIOUS DISEASES

Notification rates for children under 15 years per 100,000 population for certain infectious diseases—1951–1974

Table D.4

England and Wales

Disease	1951	1961	1966	1967	1968	1969	1970	1971	1972	1973	1974
Dysentery (amoebic and bacillary)	195·28	130·93	133·20	133·22	120·47	132·47	59·06	60·52	47·48	41·35	44·82
Food poisoning	22·73	29·77	13·85	18·51	19·24	23·44	23·24	20·17	16·68	20·12	17·59
Tuberculosis											
respiratory	..	16·29	10·76	10·33	10·19	8·63	8·00	8·57	7·90	7·70	7·50
meninges and central nervous system	..	0·75	0·37	0·37	0·34	0·30	0·35	0·34	0·27	0·19	0·21
other	..	3·28	1·66	1·81	1·72	1·97	1·95	2·05	1·91	1·91	2·24
Whooping cough	1,707·72	224·62	171·83	290·55	148·38	41·93	140·36	140·12	17·27	20·47	136·41
Scarlet fever	465·45	178·35	182·48	163·18	122·52	130·38	105·81	99·52	89·77	95·54	81·59
Acute meningitis[1]	10·91	4·98	2·96	2·04	3·95	7·61	8·20	10·09	9·30	13·51	14·27
meningococcus	..	..	..	..	..	..	3·63	3·59	4·18	7·19	8·94
other specified organisms ...	..	..	..	..	..	..	2·22	3·70	2·59	2·79	2·87
unspecified organisms ...	..	..	..	..	..	..	2·35	2·81	2·54	3·53	2·45
Measles	6,200·81	7,106·28	3,065·76	4,042·37	2,042·89	1,211·99	2,619·87	1,138·35	1,229·41	1,280·95	927·81
Acute encephalitis											
infective	1·30	0·65	0·40	0·44	0·48	0·58	0·51	0·38	0·29	0·46	0·28
post-infectious	0·81	1·09	0·74	0·78	0·41	0·65	0·74	0·31	0·57	0·43	0·24
Infective jaundice[2]	..	..	..	..	..	122·74	106·40	63·51	51·51	30·68	27·48

Source: OPCS

[1]Prior to 1 October 1968 the notifiable disease was "Meningococcal infection".
[2]Became notifiable on 15 June 1968.

INFECTIOUS DISEASES

Notification rates per 100,000 population for certain infectious diseases by sex and age group—1974

Table D.5

England and Wales

| Age group | Dysentery (amoebic and bacillary) | | Diphtheria | | Scarlet fever | | Acute meningitis due to infection with: | | | | | |
| | | | | | | | Meningococcus | | Other specified organisms | | Unspecified organisms | |
	M	F	M	F	M	F	M	F	M	F	M	F
0–14 years ...	46·52	43·03	0·02	—	78·93	84·40	9·90	7·94	3·29	2·43	2·95	1·93
Under 1 year	73·47	70·33	—	—	13·05	12·20	54·64	37·89	16·39	9·31	9·71	7·06
1–2 years	85·64	87·23	—	—	27·70	23·98	23·74	21·58	7·07	6·59	5·09	2·40
2–3 years	97·70	100·03	—	—	61·42	65·93	21·71	13·52	3·97	4·51	3·18	2·25
3–4 years	101·52	89·48	—	—	104·81	95·33	16·71	15·93	3·54	3·19	4·05	3·19
4–5 years	74·19	64·69	—	—	162·39	167·76	10·12	7·68	2·08	1·10	3·11	2·74
5–9 years	42·71	38·71	—	—	122·53	138·54	3·97	3·96	2·15	1·60	2·69	1·70
10–14 years	13·45	11·36	0·05	—	36·76	37·01	2·58	2·15	1·69	1·15	1·44	0·79

| Age group | Measles | | Acute poliomyelitis | | | | Acute encephalitis | | | |
| | | | Paralytic | | Non-paralytic | | Infective | | Post-infectious | |
	M	F	M	F	M	F	M	F	M	F
0–14 years ...	923·99	931·84	0·02	0·02	—	—	0·37	0·18	0·25	0·23
Under 1 year	739·53	761·72	0·30	—	—	—	0·30	0·32	—	0·32
1–2 years	1,565·86	1,514·39	—	—	—	—	0·28	0·90	0·28	—
2–3 years	1,467·04	1,448·01	—	0·28	—	—	0·79	—	0·53	0·28
3–4 years	1,645·32	1,661·98	—	—	—	—	0·51	—	—	0·27
4–5 years	1,876·26	1,921·05	—	—	—	—	0·52	—	0·52	1·10
5–9 years	1,232·04	1,252·42	—	—	—	—	0·54	0·26	0·39	0·26
10–14 years	104·14	103·03	—	—	—	—	0·10	0·05	0·10	0·05

Typhoid, Paratyphoid fever and Food poisoning

Age group	Typhoid fever				Paratyphoid fever				Food poisoning	
	Abroad		Presumed contracted in GB		Abroad		in GB			
	M	F	M	F	M	F	M	F	M	F
0–14 years... ...	0·42	0·16	0·14	0·09	0·14	0·09	0·08	0·09	18·66	16·45
0–4 years... ...	0·43	0·06	0·05	0·23	0·16	0·11	0·11	0·23	34·54	29·81
5–14 years... ...	0·42	0·21	0·17	0·03	0·12	0·08	0·07	0·03	11·46	10·41

Tuberculosis and Infective jaundice

Age group	Respiratory		Meninges and CNS		Other		Infective jaundice	
	M	F	M	F	M	F	M	F
0–19 years ...	8·74	8·83	0·20	0·21	2·83	2·65	24·65	27·79
Under 1 year ...	3·64	4·50	0·30	1·28	1·52	—	3·34	1·61
1–2 years ...	6·50	5·70	0·28	0·30	1·41	1·20	2·54	2·70
2–4 years ...	9·07	9·03	0·26	0·18	2·76	2·92	16·23	18·79
5–9 years ...	6·42	7·41	0·10	0·10	2·20	2·11	38·74	43·86
10–14 years ...	7·89	8·17	0·20	0·21	1·93	2·88	27·44	27·96
15–19 years ...	13·53	12·47	0·22	0·12	5·11	3·59	19·15	24·77

Whooping cough

Age group	M	F
0–14 years ...	126·21	147·16
Under 3 months[1]	45·54	53·31
3–5 months[1]	85·91	84·78
6–8 months[1]	114·45	115·93
9–11 months[1]	84·70	94·73
1–2 years ...	214·25	245·20
2–4 years ...	216·37	267·35
5–9 years ...	130·81	152·96
10–14 years ...	20·89	22·30

[1] Rates are calculated on the population aged under one year.

Source: OPCS

101

PERCENTAGE OF CHILDREN WITH DENTAL DISEASE—1973

Table D.6

PERCENTAGE OF CHILDREN

Age	No known decay experience	Active decay requiring treatment	Periodontal Disease				Orthodontic Need		Needing some dental attention
			Inflammation of gums	Debris on teeth	Calculus on teeth	Some inflammation, debris or calculus	Some treatment	Appliance therapy	
5	29	63	26	39	5	47	17	8	79
6	20	69	35	48	5	58	28	15	87
7	14	73	50	62	9	72	48	31	94
8	9	78	56	67	15	78	57	40	97
9	7	76	56	67	17	78	55	38	96
10	7	69	56	65	21	76	50	35	95
11	5	66	59	65	26	80	46	34	95
12	5	61	57	64	28	78	37	28	94
13	5	61	55	59	31	75	30	22	90
14	4	62	54	56	33	74	28	19	90
15	3	57	51	51	34	71	27	20	88

Source: Children's Dental Health in England and Wales, 1973
(J. E. Todd—HMSO, 1975)

INDIVIDUAL DENTAL DISEASE AND TREATMENT EXPERIENCE BY AGE—1973

Table D.7   England and Wales

Age	Average number of teeth with known decay experience (D,M,F and d,f) (A)	Percentage of children with active decay requiring treatment	Average number of decayed teeth per child examined (B)	Average number of decayed teeth per child with active caries (D and d)	% total decay untreated (ie active caries) (B÷A×100)	Average number of filled teeth per child examined (F and f) (C)	% total decay treated by conservation (C÷A×100)
5	3·4	63	2·6	4·1	76	0·7	21
6	3·9	69	2·7	3·9	69	1·1	28
7	4·3	73	2·8	3·8	65	1·5	35
8	5·0	78	2·8	3·6	56	2·1	42
9	5·0	76	2·5	3·3	50	2·4	48
10	4·9	69	2·1	3·0	43	2·4	49
11	4·9	66	1·9	2·9	39	2·6	53
12	5·2	61	1·7	2·8	33	3·0	58
13	6·2	61	1·7	2·8	27	3·9	63
14	7·4	62	1·9	3·1	26	4·8	65
15	8·4	57	1·6	2·8	19	6·0	71

D, M, F   mean number of permanent teeth decayed, missing or filled.
d, f   mean number of primary teeth decayed or filled.

Source: Derived from data in " Children's Dental Health in England and Wales, 1973 " (J. E. Todd—HMSO, 1975).

IN-PATIENTS, NHS NON-PSYCHIATRIC HOSPITALS
SPECIAL CARE BABIES DEPARTMENTS
ESTIMATED NUMBERS OF DISCHARGES AND DEATHS: AVERAGE DAILY BEDS—BY SEX AND DIAGNOSIS—1973

By Diagnostic Group from all Departments

England and Wales

Table D.8

List A/ ICD Number	Diagnostic group	Estimated numbers			Average beds daily			Special care infants as percentage of all infants aged under one year by discharges in all Departments
		Total	Males	Females	Total	Males	Females	
A1–150	All causes	106,230	57,630	48,600	2,810	1,445	1,365	49·5
A62–66	Endocrine, nutritional and metabolic diseases ...	1,760	1,040	720	45	30	16	21·3
251	Disorders of pancreatic internal secretion other than diabetes	440	240	200	12	7	4	85·9
269	Other nutritional deficiency	1,070	620	450	27	17	10	17·1
A126–130	Congenital anomalies	4,530	2,540	1,990	101	55	46	23·5
741	Spina bifida	630	350	280	6	3	3	27·9
746	Congenital anomalies of heart	730	370	370	18	8	10	25·9
752	Congenital anomalies of genital organs ...	320	290	20	4	3	—	53·6
755	Other congenital anomalies of limbs ...	990	370	620	14	6	8	41·0
A131–135	Certain causes of perinatal morbidity	74,370	40,010	34,360	2,252	1,146	1,106	94·1

104

Code	Cause						%
768	Difficult labour with other and unspecified complications	2,670	1,440	1,230	24	13	11	99·5
769	Other complications of pregnancy	2,010	1,050	960	88	51	37	99·3
771	Conditions of umbilical cord	480	220	260	7	2	4	89·5
772	Birth injury without mention of cause	4,510	2,660	1,850	67	39	28	96·6
775	Haemolytic disease of new-born without mention of kernicterus	2,390	1,280	1,110	32	25	57	90·7
776	Anoxic and hypoxic conditions not otherwise specified ...	15,190	9,040	6,160	306	183	123	96·3
777	Immaturity, unqualified	29,790	14,520	15,270	1,405	664	741	97·5
778	Other conditions of foetus or newborn	14,520	8,270	6,260	261	142	119	84·3
A136–137	Symptoms and ill-defined conditions	19,010	10,440	8,570	276	146	130	64·0
780	Certain symptoms referable to nervous system	460	290	170	10	6	4	12·8
784	Symptoms referable to the upper gastro-intestinal tract	460	240	220	8	4	4	15·9
788	Other general symptoms	980	660	320	18	13	5	37·4
793	Observation, without need of further medical care ...	15,740	8,460	7,280	197	96	101	94·3
796	Other ill-defined causes of morbidity and mortality ...	700	380	320	30	21	9	43·8
Remainder	Other causes	6,570	3,610	2,960	136	68	67	6·0

Source: DHSS
Hospital In-Patient Enquiry

IN-PATIENTS, NHS NON-PSYCHIATRIC HOSPITALS
PAEDIATRIC DEPARTMENTS—DISCHARGES AND DEATHS
ESTIMATED NUMBERS: AVERAGE BEDS DAILY—BY SEX AND DIAGNOSIS—1973

All discharges from Paediatric Departments as a percentage of child discharges 0–14 years from all Departments

Table D.9

England and Wales

ICD Numbers	Diagnostic group	Estimated numbers			Average beds occupied daily			Percentages of child discharges from all Departments
		Total	Males	Females	Total	Males	Females	
A1–150	All causes	245,980	144,930	101,050	4,909	2,843	2,066	27·4
A1–44 009	Infective and parasitic diseases ... Diarrhoeal diseases	23,220 11,490	13,850 6,840	9,370 4,650	474 211	293 130	181 81	51·3 52·1
A62–66	Endocrine, nutritional and metabolic diseases	13,100	6,970	6,130	453	248	205	74·8
A72–74	Diseases of the nervous system	8,830	4,970	3,870	344	195	149	68·9
A89–96 A89–90	Diseases of the respiratory system Acute respiratory infections and influenza	68,820 33,420	42,090 20,140	26,730 13,280	1,063 446	626 260	437 186	36·3 67·1
A97–104	Diseases of the digestive system ...	10,440	6,680	3,750	210	130	80	13·7
A126–130	Congenital anomalies	9,530	5,970	3,550	507	311	196	14·5
A136, 137	Symptoms and ill-defined conditions ...	37,070	20,990	16,080	559	305	254	40·1
A138–142	Fractures, dislocations and sprains ...	1,410	920	490	32	24	8	4·4
A143–150 A149	Other injuries and reactions ... ... Adverse effects of chemical substances	37,340 26,320	21,830 14,750	15,520 11,560	289 95	157 55	132 40	32·2 88·4
Remainder	Other causes	36,220	20,660	15,560	978	554	424	5·3

Source: DHSS
Hospital In-Patient Enquiry

see page 108 for Table 10

IN-PATIENTS, NHS NON-PSYCHIATRIC HOSPITALS
DISCHARGE RATES PER 10,000 POPULATION FOR SELECTED DIAGNOSES

By sex and age groups 0–19—1973
Comparison with 1968 for 0–19 only

Table D.10

England and Wales

Diagnostic group List A ICD Nos.		Rates							Index (1968 =100)	Numbers	
		Under 1 Year	1–4	5–9	10–12	13–14	15–19	0–19		1968 0–19	1973 0–19
All causes A1–150	M	3,013	888	780	527	445	509	771	102	571,660	594,030
	F	2,387	580	552	405	411	1,278	770	105	529,000	563,700
Infective and parasitic diseases A1–44	M	257	59	20	13	11	14	36	91	29,640	27,550
	F	203	43	16	9	10	18	29	87	24,180	21,180
Infections of alimentary tract A1–5	M	200	37	6	4	3	2	20	102	14,580	15,160
	F	157	25	5	2	1	2	15	86	12,170	10,680
Diseases of ear and mastoid process A78, 79 pt ...	M	28	28	63	21	16	8	31	129	17,980	23,550
	F	18	16	49	19	12	7	24	131	13,180	17,380
Otitis media and mastoiditis A78	M	27	21	31	10	9	4	17	129	10,050	13,170
	F	16	14	23	10	5	3	13	131	6,900	9,210
Diseases of respiratory system A89–96	M	368	193	226	70	41	41	141	80	132,730	108,700
	F	273	125	192	82	61	65	123	78	113,980	90,080
Acute respiratory infections and influenza A89–90	M	224	72	32	11	5	3	36	84	32,570	28,020
	F	169	48	27	10	9	9	29	84	25,100	21,350
Hypertrophy of tonsils and adenoids A94	M	1	49	149	30	14	12	59	71	62,430	45,340
	F	1	32	135	54	36	38	64	72	63,460	46,470
Diseases of digestive system A97–104	M	174	68	64	79	73	73	75	94	60,710	58,010
	F	49	28	43	66	77	94	59	97	43,680	42,890
Appendicitis A100	M	1	4	27	53	51	41	31	94	24,630	23,650
	F	—	4	22	41	50	51	29	89	24,000	21,520
Hernia (with or without obstruction) A101a ...	M	123	47	19	5	3	6	23	83	20,780	17,500
	F	15	11	6	2	1	1	5	85	4,420	3,770

108

Congenital anomalies	...	M	278	61	57	58	24	12	55	113	36,710	42,130
A126–130	...	F	205	49	25	21	22	14	34	112	21,900	24,830
Spina bifida and hydrocephalus		M	35	5	3	1	1	1	4	97	2,940	2,910
A126, 130f	...	F	33	5	3	2	1	1	4	100	2,850	2,750
Certain causes of perinatal morbidity		M	1,050	1	·	·	·	·	49	152	24,200	37,500
A131–135	...	F	940	1	·	·	·	·	43	144	21,640	31,700
Symptoms and ill-defined conditions		M	408	76	59	57	44	44	73	139	39,880	56,540
A136–137	...	F	338	58	48	55	50	82	72	142	36,670	52,890
Fractures, dislocations and sprains		M	18	23	37	40	47	72	42	98	32,700	32,730
A138–142	...	F	16	16	21	20	19	17	18	106	12,640	13,500
Other injuries and reactions	...	M	81	180	102	84	82	138	120	111	82,030	92,630
A143–150	...	F	70	134	57	43	51	96	79	120	47,840	58,110
Intra-cranial injury	...	M	32	48	59	51	39	62	53	122	33,080	40,920
A143	...	F	21	34	31	22	18	24	27	124	15,730	19,760
Adverse effects of chemical substances		M	14	82	7	3	7	25	26	127	15,490	20,010
A149	...	F	19	65	5	3	17	53	30	139	15,340	21,570

Source: DHSS
Hospital In-Patient Enquiry

109

IN-PATIENTS, NHS NON-PSYCHIATRIC HOSPITALS
AVERAGE DAILY BED RATES PER MILLION POPULATION FOR SELECTED DIAGNOSES

By sex and age groups 0–19—1973
Comparison with 1968 for 0–19 only

Table D.11

England and Wales

Diagnostic group List A ICD Nos.	Sex	Rates							Index (1968 =100)	Numbers	
		Under 1 year	1–4	5–9	10–12	13–14	15–19	0–19		1968 0–19	1973 0–19
All causes A1–150	M	7,724	1,318	1,240	916	841	1,083	1,429	75	14,481	11,013
	F	6,792	941	830	756	808	2,210	1,426	86	11,940	10,437
Infective and parasitic diseases A1–44	M	696	114	62	31	29	63	94	58	1,233	724
	F	564	88	36	27	29	83	79	63	914	579
Infections of alimentary tract A1–5	M	538	65	8	6	6	4	42	75	421	327
	F	413	43	8	3	3	5	32	65	356	232
Diseases of ear and mastoid process A78, 79 pt.	M	41	29	56	22	23	12	31	94	247	241
	F	30	22	42	20	15	10	24	100	176	177
Otitis media and mastoiditis A78	M	39	22	28	11	12	8	19	90	162	143
	F	28	17	22	10	6	5	14	93	108	102
Diseases of respiratory system A89–96	M	716	231	229	90	63	72	178	64	2,094	1,373
	F	544	154	205	94	79	99	156	66	1,695	1,143
Acute respiratory infections and influenza A89–90	M	384	75	35	12	5	4	46	68	511	352
	F	294	57	29	11	12	13	38	70	392	281
Hypertrophy of tonsils and adenoids A94	M	6	46	141	30	17	18	58	67	656	446
	F	4	30	127	55	47	53	66	68	704	481
Diseases of digestive system A97–104	M	252	86	102	141	127	126	120	82	1,110	922
	F	104	39	71	102	118	143	92	77	860	671
Appendicitis A100	M	3	11	58	106	100	79	62	84	560	480
	F	2	8	47	80	92	90	57	76	540	414
Hernia (with or without obstruction) … M	142	43	21			25				

110

Diseases of musculo-skeletal system A121–125	M	28	44	76	62	99	75	67	58	880	518
	F	8	20	42	84	100	76	56	79	510	409
Congenital anomalies A126–130	M	1,186	163	142	127	52	61	165	97	1,290	1,270
	F	939	182	86	66	66	43	130	95	990	949
Spina bifida and hydrocephalus A126, 130f	M	143	15	35	12	9	5	23	88	196	177
	F	266	26	14	10	8	3	24	80	220	179
Certain causes of perinatal morbidity A131–135	M	3,041	6	..	..	..	..	141	119	890	1,090
	F	3,050	7	..	..	..	..	141	116	880	1,033
Symptoms and ill-defined conditions A136–137	M	635	88	95	65	57	52	100	108	700	773
	F	562	79	64	69	64	101	99	124	580	725
Fractures, dislocations and sprains A138–142	M	49	88	105	103	108	275	138	84	1,250	1,061
	F	25	52	52	48	74	63	41	71	422	297
Other injuries and reactions A143–150	M	163	158	111	89	107	157	129	78	1,251	998
	F	131	103	64	80	48	96	83	100	601	609
Intra-cranial injury A143	M	26	32	48	32	24	51	39	70	426	301
	F	41	18	26	43	14	34	28	140	148	206
Adverse effects of chemical substances A149	M	7	30	4	2	16	15	13	108	88	99
	F	7	23	2	2	11	35	15	136	83	107

Source: DHSS
Hospital In-Patient Enquiry

111

IN-PATIENTS, NHS NON-PSYCHIATRIC HOSPITALS
MEAN DURATION OF STAY (DAYS) FOR SELECTED DIAGNOSES

By Sex and age groups 0–19 for 1973
Comparison with 1968 for 0–19 only

Table D.12

England and Wales

Diagnosis / List A ICD Nos.	Sex	1973							1968	Index (1968 = 100)
		Under 1 year	1–4	5–9	10–12	13–14	15–19	0–19	0–19	
All causes A1–150	M	9·4	5·4	5·8	6·3	6·9	7·8	6·8	9·3	73
	F	10·4	5·9	5·5	6·8	7·2	6·3	6·7	8·3	81
Infective and parasitic diseases A1–44	M	9·9	7·1	11·4	8·5	9·3	15·8	9·6	15·2	63
	F	10·2	7·5	8·1	10·4	10·5	16·4	10·0	13·8	72
Infections of alimentary tract A5	M	9·8	6·4	5·2	6·3	4·8	6·6	7·9	10·6	75
	F	9·6	6·3	6·2	4·8	9·0	7·1	8·0	10·7	75
Diseases of the ear and mastoid process A78, A79 pt ...	M	5·4	3·7	3·2	3·8	5·3	5·9	3·7	5·0	74
	F	6·2	4·1	3·1	3·8	4·5	5·4	3·7	4·9	76
Otitis media and mastoiditis A78	M	5·4	4·0	3·3	4·1	4·7	7·1	4·0	5·9	68
	F	6·3	4·4	3·5	3·8	4·3	5·9	4·0	5·7	70
Diseases of the respiratory system A89–96	M	7·1	4·4	3·7	4·7	5·7	6·3	4·6	5·8	79
	F	7·3	4·5	3·9	4·2	4·7	5·5	4·6	5·4	85
Acute respiratory infection and influenza A89–90	M	6·3	3·8	4·1	3·8	4·1	5·0	4·6	5·7	81
	F	6·4	4·3	3·9	4·0	4·5	5·3	4·8	5·7	84
Hypertrophy of tonsils and adenoids A94	M	15·2	3·5	3·4	3·7	4·6	5·3	3·6	3·9	92
	F	10·0	3·4	3·4	3·7	4·8	5·1	3·8	4·0	95
Diseases of the digestive system A97–104	M	5·3	4·6	5·8	6·5	5·7	6·3	5·8	6·7	87
	F	7·8	5·1	6·0	5·6	5·8	5·6	5·7	7·1	

Appendicitis	M	[illegible]	[illegible]	[illegible]	[illegible]	[illegible]	[illegible]	[illegible]	[illegible]	[illegible]
A100	F	..	7·9	8·0	7·2	6·8	6·5	7·0	8·3	84
Hernia (with or without obstruction)	M	4·2	3·3	4·1	4·2	4·7	6·6	4·0	5·0	80
A101a	F	4·8	2·6	3·6	3·2	4·0	5·9	3·4	5·5	62
Diseases of the musculo-skeletal system	M	17·1	18·3	19·3	16·3	18·1	13·3	16·6	25·6	65
A121–125	F	5·8	12·1	16·0	22·0	16·6	11·1	14·6	17·8	82
Congenital anomalies	M	15·6	9·7	9·2	8·1	7·9	18·0	11·0	12·9	85
A126–130	F	16·7	13·6	12·6	11·7	14·2	11·7	14·0	16·6	84
Spina bifida and hydrocephalus	M	14·8	10·2	47·0	42·5[1]	25·4[1]	64·0	22·2	24·3	91
A126, A130f	F	29·4	18·4	18·0	21·8[1]	50·0[1]	31·5	23·8	28·1	85
Certain causes of perinatal morbidity	M	10·6	19·1	.	.	.	.	13·0	13·5	96
A131–135	F	11·8	18·3	.	.	.	.	14·5	14·9	97
Symptoms and ill-defined conditions	M	5·7	4·2	5·9	4·2	4·7	4·3	5·0	6·4	78
A136–137	F	6·1	5·0	4·9	4·5	4·6	4·5	5·0	5·8	86
Fractures, dislocations and sprains	M	9·8	14·0	10·4	9·5	8·4	14·1	11·9	14·0	85
A138–142	F	5·4	11·8	8·9	9·0	14·3	13·8	10·9	12·2	89
Other injuries and reactions	M	7·3	3·2	4·0	3·9	4·8	4·2	4·0	5·6	71
A143–150	F	6·8	2·8	4·1	6·8	3·5	3·7	3·8	4·6	83
Intra-cranial injury	M	3·0	2·4	2·9	2·3	2·2	3·1	2·7	4·8	56
A143	F	7·0	1·9	3·0	7·1	2·7	5·1	3·8	3·5	109
Adverse effects of chemical substances	M	1·8	1·3	2·3	2·1	8·3	2·2	1·8	2·1	86
A149	F	1·4	1·3	1·4	2·1	2·4	2·4	1·8	2·0	90

Source: DHSS
Hospital In-Patient Enquiry

[1]These averages are based on fewer than 20 sample cases and are subject to relatively high margins of sampling error.

CHILD MORBIDITY—NON-PSYCHIATRIC
HOSPITAL DISCHARGE RATES PER 10,000 POPULATION UNDER 15 YEARS OF AGE FOR SELECTED DIAGNOSES

By sex and Regional Hospital Board area of residence—1973

Table D.13

England and Wales

Regional Hospital Board	All Causes A1-150			Diseases of Respiratory System A89-96	Hypertrophy of Tonsils and Adenoids A94	Diseases of Digestive System A97-104	Symptoms and Ill-defined conditions A136-137	Fractures, Dislocations and Sprains A138-142	Other Injuries and reactions A143-150	Adverse effects of chemical substances A149
	Estimated numbers 1973	Rate Index (1968= 100)[1]	Rates							
MALES										
England and Wales	.	102	845·2	169·9	72·5	75·8	81·6	33·7	114·2	26·0
Estimated Numbers	503,280		.	101,190	43,190	45,120	48,600	20,110	68,010	15,480
Newcastle	30,370	99	798·9	167·4	62·0	77·7	73·6	35·8	110·0	18·6
Leeds	34,670	97	876·3	168·3	84·5	76·0	83·5	33·0	130·4	28·3
Sheffield	40,240	106	687·5	121·5	42·6	60·3	63·2	28·9	96·1	25·9
East Anglian	17,770	140	812·7	128·3	46·8	76·8	89·9	27·3	100·9	29·4
NW Metropolitan	42,640	108	891·4	184·7	73·2	75·7	95·1	33·7	108·3	24·3
NE Metropolitan	37,020	99	928·3	211·5	81·0	81·8	93·3	34·1	115·4	30·8
SE Metropolitan	37,770	117	947·6	194·7	83·2	82·9	95·5	39·7	114·9	21·3
SW Metropolitan	32,330	103	902·8	192·3	82·6	74·4	96·3	35·2	107·6	21·3
Wessex	20,060	100	795·6	177·7	107·9	62·5	87·9	35·2	108·8	20·3
Oxford	22,520	100	832·0	158·3	72·8	67·8	61·5	31·2	109·9	24·4
South Western	29,810	103	797·4	152·6	63·7	83·2	76·1	33·7	116·3	27·5
Birmingham	49,880	96	754·6	160·7	70·5	66·7	70·7	30·1	110·2	26·9
Manchester	50,240	97	897·3	187·1	95·1	91·4	77·4	31·7	121·9	26·0
Liverpool	26,650	94	908·4	161·1	47·8	76·4	79·7	36·6	120·9	26·1
Wales	21,220	110	947·5	182·3	75·7	85·2				

Region										Estimated Numbers
England and Wales	20·4	67·6	17·3	63·4	44·0	64·8	126·1	618·1	103[1]	
Estimated Numbers	12,610	41,760	10,670	39,190	27,220	40,060	77,940		[1]	349,120
Newcastle	14·6	73·0	18·9	71·5	45·0	61·8	136·9	613·5		22,300
Leeds	27·1	89·2	21·4	63·7	45·8	92·2	154·8	680·3		25,570
Sheffield	21·5	60·8	15·3	52·3	37·0	39·1	96·7	482·2		26,900
East Anglian ...	23·5	70·4	22·9	76·5	41·9	54·8	124·0	616·8		12,690
NW Metropolitan ...	21·6	71·8	19·9	86·7	48·3	72·8	149·2	660·0		29,900
NE Metropolitan ...	21·7	72·7	18·0	83·7	60·0	75·6	172·3	680·1		25,550
SE Metropolitan ...	23·4	81·0	20·2	82·4	48·6	72·6	147·8	661·6		24,900
SW Metropolitan ...	15·6	67·4	17·6	82·7	60·3	92·9	171·1	689·2		23,490
Wessex	18·1	66·1	24·0	56·3	46·0	97·4	145·3	565·8		13,490
Oxford	24·2	84·6	20·2	49·7	47·5	66·2	116·9	560·1		14,250
South Western ...	20·6	68·7	20·9	73·3	53·3	63·2	92·6	571·9		20,220
Birmingham	24·1	72·3	17·8	52·0	44·3	68·1	118·6	542·4		33,880
Manchester	23·6	73·2	16·5	67·2	52·7	84·9	160·4	661·3		35,380
Liverpool	23·6	83·1	15·2	68·2	44·2	46·9	137·6	662·8		18,470
Wales	30·8	85·1	21·2	87·9	51·1	84·4	159·9	699·9		22,130

[1] Males and females combined—1968 data by sex not available.

Source: DHSS
Hospital In-Patient Enquiry

VENEREAL DISEASES 1966–1974

New cases of primary and secondary syphilis and gonorrhoea (post-pubertal infections) by age groups and sex

Table D.14

England and Wales

	Sex	1966	1967	1968	1969	1970	1971	1972	1973	1974
New cases of primary and secondary syphilis ...	T	1,374	1,320	1,320	1,265	1,162	1,187	1,222	1,549	1,685
	M	1,132	1,074	1,085	1,043	969	963	1,030	1,329	1,425
	F	242	246	235	222	193	224	192	220	260
Aged under 16	M	5	2	3	2	2	3	1	4	3
	F	1	2	2	3	2	5	8	4	2
Aged 16–17	M	14	20	16	21	16	17	26	20	18
	F	15	16	18	20	10	12	11	14	21
Aged 18–19	M	57	72	55	61	38	54	50	64	72
	F	35	26	34	40	29	33	28	26	34
New cases of gonorrhoea (post-pubertal infections) ...	T	37,378	41,711	44,873	51,132	54,671	57,469	54,901	60,170	59,685
	M	27,913	30,630	32,586	36,364	37,784	39,031	36,071	38,871	38,442
	F	9,465	11,081	12,287	14,768	16,887	18,438	18,830	21,299	21,243
Aged under 16	M	53	41	75	83	85	131	116	153	127
	F	153	182	236	351	409	410	431	466	480
Aged 16–17	M	520	582	685	846	930	1,065	968	1,135	1,204
	F	827	1,036	1,210	1,567	1,974	2,193	2,318	2,617	2,526
Aged 18–19	M	1,973	2,295	2,526	3,126	3,292	3,473	3,302	3,673	3,614
	F	1,693	2,034	2,160	2,743	3,240	3,540	3,695	4,165	4,181

Source: DHSS
Welsh Office

CHILDREN AND YOUNG PEOPLE CONSULTING A GENERAL PRACTITIONER

Rates per 1,000 population by age and diagnosed condition—1970–1971

Table D.15

England and Wales

ICD No.	Cause	0–4	5–14	15–24
	All diseases and conditions	896·8	639·0	686·7
001–136	Infective and parasitic diseases	181·7	141·9	73·7
003–005, 007–009	Intestinal infection and disease	58·2	16·3	19·3
055	Measles	33·4	13·2	0·3
079·1	Viral warts	4·5	39·2	14·9
320–389	Diseases of the nervous system and sense organs	235·2	127·2	84·2
360	Conjunctivitis and ophthalmia	65·4	17·8	13·0
381·0	Acute otitis media	146·6	68·5	12·5
460–519	Diseases of the respiratory system	548·2	325·7	256·8
460 (pt)	Acute naso-pharyngitis nonfebrile	249·4	78·9	58·3
460 (rdr)	Acute naso-pharyngitis febrile (including sporadic influenza-like illness)	122·1	56·9	42·8
462, 463	Acute pharyngitis and acute tonsilitis	161·4	146·4	102·1
466 (pt)	Acute bronchitis and bronchiolitis	143·3	58·5	30·1
680–709	Diseases of the skin and subcutaneous tissue	176·5	127·1	139·3
691, 692·9	Other eczema and dermatitis—non-specific or unspecified (including infantile eczema)	70·7	23·1	22·5
780–796	Symptoms and ill-defined conditions	264·7	139·3	121·7
783·3	Cough	97·1	43·0	13·5
561, 784·1 (pt)	Acute vomiting and/or diarrhoea	101·7	29·2	29·7
N800–N999	Accidents, poisonings and violence	84·6	99·5	121·1
N870–N929 (rdr)	Lacerations, traumatic amputations, superficial injuries, contusions, abrasions, crushings (except insect bites)	46·5	54·5	57·0
	Prophylactic procedures and other medical examinations	270·0	60·4	216·2

Source: OPCS
Morbidity Statistics from General Practice
Second National Study 1970–1971

ATTENDANCE ALLOWANCES IN PAYMENT ON 1 DECEMBER 1972 AND 30 JUNE 1974 IN RESPECT OF CHILDREN AND YOUNG PEOPLE AGED 2-19

Analysed by age group, sex and Social Security Administrative Region[1]

Table D.16   England and Wales

MALES

Social Security Administrative Region[1]	Children aged 2-15			Young people aged 16-19		
	1.12.72	Allowances current on 30.6.74		1.12.72	Allowances current on 30.6.74	
	Higher Rate	Higher Rate	Lower Rate	Higher Rate	Higher Rate	Lower Rate
England and Wales	10,736	11,670	5,474	1,168	1,485	1,143
Northern	884	968	330	94	125	81
Yorkshire and Humberside ...	1,087	1,260	536	129	163	136
East Midlands and East Anglia ...	1,104	1,164	569	144	191	115
London	3,176	3,598	1,557	283	385	311
GLC offices	1,203	1,314	417	112	162	98
Non-GLC offices	1,973	2,284	1,140	171	223	213
South Western	668	741	410	72	92	91
West Midlands	1,142	1,204	753	111	157	147
North Western	2,063	2,060	905	237	265	180

England and Wales	8,360	9,074	4,287	973	1,237	1,031
Northern	661	719	260	65	104	75
Yorkshire and Humberside ...	837	941	451	93	137	122
East Midlands and East Anglia ...	928	978	449	127	146	108
London	2,534	2,831	1,292	275	338	282
GLC offices	995	1,061	339	100	134	96
Non-GLC offices	1,539	1,770	953	175	204	186
South Western	544	579	300	59	80	75
West Midlands	788	864	575	94	112	122
North Western	1,550	1,596	682	181	220	177
Wales	518	566	278	79	100	70

[1] Social Security Administrative Regions are very similar to but not identical with Standard Regions.

Source: DHSS

ATTENDANCE ALLOWANCES IN PAYMENT ON 30 JUNE 1974 IN RESPECT OF CHILDREN AND YOUNG PEOPLE AGED 2–19

Analysed by main cause of helplessness, age group and sex

Table D.17   England and Wales

Rate allowance: H=Higher   L=Lower

Age group		2–19		2–4		5–9		10–14		15		16–19		Rate per 100,000 population aged 2–19	
		H	L	H	L	H	L	H	L	H	L	H	L	H	L
Main causes of helplessness by Section of ICD 1965															
I to X and XII to XVII ...	T	23,466	11,935	3,502	2,917	9,446	3,425	6,806	2,916	990	503	2,722	2,174	172·0	87·5
All causes[1] ...	M	13,155	6,617	1,878	1,607	5,329	1,990	3,930	1,597	533	280	1,485	1,143	188·0	94·6
	F	10,311	5,318	1,624	1,310	4,117	1,435	2,876	1,319	457	223	1,237	1,031	155·1	80·0
I Infective and parasitic diseases	T	114	41	15	5	52	8	26	15	6	3	15	10	0·8	0·3
	M	45	15	6	2	23	3	11	7	1	1	4	2	0·6	0·2
	F	69	26	9	3	29	5	15	8	5	2	11	8	1·0	0·4
II Neoplasms ...	T	103	70	12	22	48	16	19	16	7	4	17	12	0·8	0·5
	M	55	38	6	12	23	11	14	8	4	1	8	6	0·8	0·5
	F	48	32	6	10	25	5	5	5	3	3	9	6	0·7	0·5
III Endocrine, nutritional and metabolic diseases	T	317	198	50	67	128	80	101	36	10	3	28	12	2·3	1·5
	M	186	99	39	31	65	42	58	16	8	3	16	7	2·7	1·4
	F	131	99	11	36	63	38	43	20	2	—	12	5	2·0	1·5
V Mental disorders ...	T	7,035	4,248	783	739	2,757	1,232	2,198	1,126	368	223	929	928	51·6	31·1
	M	4,110	2,501	476	446	1,601	774	1,325	662	192	125	516	494	58·7	35·7
	F	2,925	1,747	307	293	1,156	458	873	464	176	98	413	434	44·0	26·3

Numbers

VI Diseases of the nervous system and sense organs ...	T	6,253	2,093	901	724	2,304	1,832	603	418	261	90	855	266		17·2
	M	3,625	1,204	492	415	1,382	1,096	362	239	149	32	506	156	51·8	17·2
	F	2,628	889	409	309	1,022	736	241	179	112	28	349	132	39·5	13·4
VII Diseases of the circulatory system ...	T	100	50	25	15	38	25	16	13	3	—	9	6	0·7	0·4
	M	59	25	17	7	24	14	9	7	2	—	2	2	0·8	0·4
	F	41	25	8	8	14	11	7	6	1	—	7	4	0·6	0·4
X Diseases of the genito-urinary system ...	T	46	58	10	2	19	12	7	14	1	6	4	29	0·3	0·4
	M	25	39	7	1	10	6	5	8	1	5	1	20	0·4	0·6
	F	21	19	3	1	9	6	2	6	—	1	3	9	0·3	0·3
XIII Diseases of the musculo-skeletal system and connective tissue ...	T	191	217	30	42	96	40	124	31	2	6	23	14	1·4	1·6
	M	111	141	21	27	65	19	92	20	—	2	6	0	1·6	2·0
	F	80	76	9	15	31	21	32	11	2	4	17	14	1·2	1·1
XIV Congenital anomalies ...	T	8,188	4,545	1,494	1,290	3,492	2,226	1,208	1,156	290	186	686	805	60·0	33·3
	M	4,294	2,305	709	596	1,890	1,200	608	576	152	107	343	418	61·4	32·9
	F	3,894	2,240	785	594	1,602	1,026	600	580	138	79	343	387	58·6	33·7
XVII Accidents, poisonings and violence ...	T	151	96	22	4	43	54	27	34	8	5	24	26	1·1	0·7
	M	96	63	12	3	31	32	20	22	5	1	16	17	1·4	0·9
	F	55	33	10	1	12	22	7	12	3	4	8	9	0·8	0·5
IV, VIII, IX, XII, XV and XVI Other causes[1] ...	T	968	319	160	107	369	273	104	57	34	7	132	44	7·1	2·3
	M	549	187	93	67	215	155	64	32	19	3	67	21	7·8	2·7
	F	419	132	67	40	154	118	40	25	15	4	65	23	6·3	2·0
All causes:— Rate[2] per 100,000 population in the age group ...	M	188·0	94·6	162·0	138·7	261·0	194·9	97·5	79·2	142·1	74·7	105·6	81·3	· ·	· ·
	F	155·1	80·0	148·0	119·4	212·0	150·6	73·9	69·1	128·4	62·6	92·2	76·8	· ·	· ·

[1] Section XI is omitted as it is inappropriate to attendance allowance.

[2] Rate calculated using OPCS estimates for mid-1974 for England and Wales.

Source: DHSS

121

Section E

HEALTH AND PERSONAL SOCIAL SERVICES

This section covers the use of services by children.

There are four parts dealing respectively with community-based health services, personal social services, the acute hospitals, and mental health services for children and adolescents.

Preventive Health and Community Care

Tables E.1 and 2 are about child health centres, E.1 providing information on the number and type of premises in use and E.2 on the number of children attending and the number of sessions held. E.1 shows that the number of premises used has fallen since 1972 and that the reduction has occurred through decreased use of buildings such as church halls. The use of recognised health centres has, however, increased rapidly from 266 in 1971 to 621 in 1974. A concentration of services on fewer premises is apparent although figures in E.1 cannot distinguish between Maternity and Child Health centres. Table E.2 shows the number of children attending these centres each year. It will be noted that total attendances have declined but this is not surprising since the birth rate has fallen continuously since 1964. A greater proportion of children have been seen at child health clinics in recent years and there has in fact been very little change between 1971 and 1974 in the number of sessions. Since 1964 there has been a marked increase in the number of sessions held by health visitors and, on a much smaller scale, by hospital medical staff.

Table E.3 provides information for the three years 1971 to 1973 by hospital region on the proportion of children born two years previously who had been protected against whooping cough, diphtheria, poliomyelitis, tetanus and measles by vaccination or immunisation. Although there was some slight improvement in the national proportions vaccinated between 1971 and 1973, there were marked regional variations. Liverpool and Manchester stand out as the regions where the proportion of children vaccinated is lowest. Measles vaccination, which is of more recent origin, is much lower in most regions than vaccination against whooping cough, diphtheria, tetanus and polio but even this covered 70% of the children under 2 in the Wessex and Oxford regions in 1973.

Because of the change in administrative regions on the reorganisation of the NHS on 1 April 1974, regional data for 1974 is not available. However, the national figures for 1974 indicate that the proportion of children being vaccinated is decreasing slightly. The proportion of children born in 1972 and vaccinated by 1974 in England and Wales is as follows: diphtheria 80%, whooping cough 77%, poliomyelitis 79%, tetanus 80% and measles 52%.

Very little is known on a regular basis about the contacts between general practitioners and children. Section D provided some information on child morbidity seen by general practitioners, derived from the National Morbidity Study of 1970–71. Table E.4 provides further information on the annual patient consulting and consultation rate for children, distinguishing separately those consultations for vaccination and inoculation. The annual patient consulting rate for children is very high, 897 per 1,000 for children aged 0–4. Put another way, this means that 10% of children aged 0–4 do not see a general practitioner in a year. Patients consulting rates fall sharply with age and the rate for children aged 5–14 is 639 per 1,000. As mentioned in section D comparison of the 1955–56 and 1970–71 surveys suggests that the proportion of children not consulting a gp has increased in a year—from just under 25% to about 28% but there is no way of assessing the extent to which telephone contacts with parents and health visitor contacts have compensated for this.

Table E.7 from the same survey shows the rate of referral from general practitioner to hospital, in-patient, out-patient or for investigation only. About 12% of children aged 0–14 are referred, mostly to out-patient departments (5%) or for investigations (5%).

Tables E.5 and 6 provide data on child contacts with general practitioners derived from the General Household Survey. This data is based on self-reported consultations within the past two weeks for those interviewed. For consultations per person at risk per year it compares quite well with the 1971 National Morbidity Study—recording, however, slightly more consultations with the 0–4 age group than did the NMS, 4·2 in 1971 compared with 3·6 for the NMS. But this was probably due to differences in design which are fully discussed in the 1972 GHS report. Table E.5 also shows the breakdown between consultations at home, at the surgery and by telephone. About a quarter of consultations for children aged 0–4 take place at home but this falls to 17% for the 5–14s. E.6 shows the extent of regional variations and average consultations per child per year for 1971/72 combined. Generally speaking, the average is higher in the North of England and in Wales than in the rest of England.

Table E.8 provides information on community health dental services for children under five years of age and shows that attendance rates have increased marginally up to 1973 with a slight falling off in 1974. The rates, in any case, are very low and the 61,000 courses of treatment must be set against the nearly 1 million provided by the General Dental Service in 1974.

Table E.9 provides information for the period 1964–74 on the number of school children inspected by medical and dental officers and the numbers found to require some treatment. The emphasis will change from year to year depending on the age structure of school children. The table shows that fewer visual and hearing defects are discovered now than 10 years ago but in more recent years a greater number of children were considered to be in need of guidance and speech therapy.

The Personal Social Services

This section deals with the services for children administered by Social Services Departments of Local Authorities.

The figures in Table E.10 show the growth of recognised children's day care facilities for the last four years. Registered premises include nurseries attached to factories, etc. as well as most playgroups; registered persons are mostly childminders working in their own homes. The number of children attending at any one time may well be different from these figures of registrations. Over this period there have also developed a large number of unregistered child-minders, who have not been included in these figures.

The figures in Table E.11 show the growth of the number of children in care in recent years. These children may be in care on account of family circumstances alone, or because of a care or court order. The principal reason for the children coming into care is given in Table E.12; the distribution for children in care would be different because children admitted for short term illness or the confinement of the mother, for instance, would tend to stay for a shorter period than those admitted under a care order.

Table E.13 sets out the analysis of the registration rate for children under 16 on the local authority registers of blind and partially sighted children, deaf and hard of hearing children, and children on the general classes register of handicapped persons. A considerable effort has been made in recent years to persuade people to register, so that much of the change, particularly for the general classes register, will be due to changes in registration practice rather than changes in the number of handicapped children. Moreover, registration is voluntary and not all those entitled to be registered, even in recent years, in fact take advantage of that opportunity. The blind registers are probably more complete than those for other handicaps, but even here they are not likely to be entirely accurate.

The Hospital Services

Tables E.14–16 provide basic time series on hospital in-patient activity for children, by age. These are derived from the Hospital In-patient Enquiry (HIPE)—an analysis of 10% of hospital discharges and deaths in non-psychiatric hospitals. Discharge rates for all categories of patient have increased since 1960 and those for children are no exception—the increase has been most rapid for children under one year of age, which reflects not only the increasing tendency for children to be born in hospital but also the expansion of special care baby units. Discharge rates for ages 1–4 have also increased but less dramatically than for babies. Otherwise, discharge rates have not fluctuated much; an interesting trend however is the increase for girls aged 15–19 which reflects the increase in accidental poisoning.

Over the same period the average number of occupied beds per 1,000 children has steadily fallen except for children under one where the provision has increased slightly since 1946. Overall, however, the average number of occupied beds per 1,000 children is now two-thirds of the 1964 figure for both boys and girls, and in 1973 amounted to 11,000 for boys and 8,400 for girls (not including maternity). The fall in bed use coupled with, if anything, a slight overall increase in discharge rates has been achieved by significant reductions in average length of stay set out in Table E.16. For both boys and girls, mean length of stay has fallen by nearly 40% from 11·1 days for boys aged 0–14 in 1960 to 6·6 days in 1973; and from 11·8 in 1960 to 7·0 in 1973 for girls. The fall has been greatest for older children.

Table E.17 sets out the change in the pattern of duration of stay in somewhat more detail for 1973 compared with 1962 and shows that there has been a marked increase in discharges of the 0–4 age group for periods of a week and less, and a marked reduction in discharge of children aged 5–14 after periods of a month or more. The change in pattern may reflect not only a genuine reduction in mean durations for a given condition but possibly also a greater readiness to admit children to hospital for short periods.

Table E.18 analyses discharges and discharge rates for boys and girls by hospital department for 1973. Paediatric and special care baby departments account for over half the cases aged 0–4, but only 17% of cases aged 5–14 were dealt with in paediatric departments. For that age group general surgery, ear, nose and throat, and traumatic and orthopaedic departments accounted for over 60% of both girls and boys.

E.19 compares discharge rates for 1960 and 1973 for boys and girls in the two main age groups for each of the hospital regions. Although the general pattern of change is consistent, in that discharge rates have increased for 0–4s and either fallen or stayed about the same for 5–14s, the actual discharge rates vary considerably from region to region. For boys aged 0–4, for example, the range is from 967 per 10,000 in Sheffield to 1,525 in Liverpool (the England and Wales average was 1,285 in 1973).

Tables E.20, 21 and 22 provide information on the beds available in paediatric departments, infectious diseases departments and special care baby units. They are derived from the SH3 return, the general statistical return completed by all hospitals. E.20 classifies the 325 paediatric departments in England in 1973 by region and number of beds showing that 79 had less than 10 beds and 204 less than 24. A similar classification of the 120 infectious diseases departments is given in E.21. By contrast much more information is given in E.22 about the 275 special care baby units in England and Wales. The average daily number of available cots has increased from 2,510 in 1964 to 4,210 in 1975, the high increase in discharges noted earlier being facilitated partly by a fall in mean duration of stay from 13·3 days in 1964 to 8·8 in 1975. There has been considerable regional variation in the extent to which this change has taken place. It is clear that there is no uniformity about admission to special care units and average length of stay from one unit to another.

Table E.23 shows the number of discharges from two regional centres, Newcastle AHA(T) and the Great Ormond Street Hospital for Sick Children, by diagnostic group compared with the national totals.

Table E.24 provides statistics from the SH3 return on day cases and out-patient attendances in paediatric departments. All the indicators of hospital out-patient activity have increased; clinic sessions have increased from 37,291 in 1964 to 69,864 in 1975 and the number of new out-patients rose steadily from 131,000 in 1954 and 149,000 in 1964 to 199,000 in 1974. Attendances per out-patient have increased from 4·2 in 1964 to 5·4 in 1974. Consequently, total attendances have increased more rapidly than new out-patients and the implication is that rather fewer patients are now seen per session. Part (b) of the table

125

sets out the changes between 1964 and 1972 in paediatric out-patient attendances by Regional Hospital Board while part (c) gives figures for Regional Health Authorities in 1974 and 1975.

There is no regular comprehensive statistical information on the characteristics of out-patients—the breakdown and any changes in the pattern by age, sex and diagnosis are unknown. The same is true of accident and emergency departments, which inevitably deal with a large number of children as casualties each year. These aspects of hospital service for children cannot be measured precisely. The next two tables, E.25 and 26, provide some information about accident and emergency departments from special enquiries while tables E.27–29 give the results of special analyses of accident and emergency activity for children at three hospitals with special information systems. The results of these cannot of course be extrapolated to describe the national situation with any certainty but provide a possible clue to the pattern. Finally in this group, Table E.30 sets out for 1973 an analysis of the children treated as out-patients in the Royal Chesterfield Hospital where a feasibility trial of out-patient activity analysis has been in operation for some years.

Mental Health

The final group of tables, E.31–37, cover the treatment of children and adolescents in mental illness and mental handicap hospitals and units. Table E.31 shows that a very small proportion of the resident in-patients of mental illness hospitals are children under 15 (5% in 1971) although the number has increased threefold since 1954. Adolescents aged 15–19 resident as in-patients account for a higher proportion (10% in 1971), but the number of adolescents has declined slightly since 1963 as alternative services have developed and more in-patient care is given on a short stay basis.

Table E.32 summarises hospital services specifically for child psychiatry (including child guidance) over the period 1964–1974. Both numbers of available beds and discharges have increased but there are marked regional variations in the levels of service provided. Out-patient activities increased over the decade, but it should be noted that the "attendances" statistics which refer to contacts with the patient only may underestimate the total volume of work and the rate of growth, particularly as discussions with parents, relatives and others are excluded and may have increased considerably in recent years.

Table E.33, which gives similar information for adolescent psychiatry units for 1972–74, shows that both in-patient and out-patient services have expanded rapidly and that, again, there are marked regional variations.

Table E.34 analyses admissions of children and adolescents to mental illness hospitals and units between 1964 and 1974. Admission rates for children under 5 are low, 5 per 100,000, but they have doubled since 1964. For the older children and adolescents the admission rates are higher and although they have increased since 1964 there have been no marked changes since 1970 apart from a slight decline for adolescents, particularly in 1974. Rates for girls aged 15 to 19 are over a third higher than the rates for boys of the same age, but in the 5–9 age

126

group, the girls' admission rate is only half that for boys. The rates are approximately the same for both boys and girls in other groups. Although not strictly comparable over the whole period, first admissions (Table E.35) for children under 15 increased from 1964 to 1974. Nevertheless, first admission rates since 1970 show little change for children and a slow decline for adolescents aged 15–19 which was most noticeable in 1974.

Tables E.36 and 37 provide some information on children in mental handicap hospitals and units. Table E.36 shows that at the end of 1974 there were over 4,600 children under 15 in mental handicap beds, considerably more than in mental illness hospitals and units but a substantial decrease on the 7,000 in mental handicap beds at the end of 1963. Again, there are considerable variations between the regions in the numbers of children accommodated as in-patients but the differences have narrowed since 1963. Table E.37 analyses admissions of children to mental handicap hospitals and units and shows that for children under 5 admission rates have declined slightly since 1964 while they have increased for older children. Over this period the practice of admitting the mentally handicapped into hospital for short periods to give respite to parents and families who normally care for them has developed and the increase in admissions for children can be attributed to this. The decline in the number of children resident on a particular day has occurred because relatively few children are now being admitted and becoming long stay in-patients.

Hospital in-patient statistics for the mentally ill and mentally handicapped cover only the most serious cases. The majority of these client groups live, and are cared for, outside hospitals and the services they receive are planned to expand to treat more of those who previously would have been cared for in hospital. In fact there are no local authority hostel places for mentally ill children and only about 1,000 mentally handicapped children are cared for in LA homes and hostels. Mental illness in children, therefore, when treated in the community, will be family-based in conjunction with general practitioners and out-patient departments.

NUMBER OF PREMISES IN USE AS MATERNITY AND CHILD HEALTH CENTRES—1964, 1971–1974

Table E.1

England and Wales

Year	Total	Health Centres[3]	Maternity and Child Health Centres[1]			Other Buildings		
			Purpose built	Adapted	Mobile	GP Surgeries (excluding those in health centres)	On a sessional basis in connection with mobile child health centres	Other premises[2] (eg. church halls) used on a sessional basis
1964	6,411	..	..	..	..	..	..	..
1971	6,608	266	1,459	758	55	298	170	3,602
1972	6,722	399	1,403	751	60	500	167	3,422
1973	6,683	507	1,393	712	47	527	164	3,333
1974	6,506	621	1,346	652	81	569	96	3,141

[1] A separate classification of premises used as child health centres is not available.
[2] Includes premises used by voluntary organisations.
[3] Only includes buildings which the Secretary of State has formally approved as health centres under Section 21 of the National Health Service Act 1946.

Source: DHSS
Welsh Office

NUMBER OF CHILDREN ATTENDING AND NUMBER OF SESSIONS HELD AT CHILD HEALTH CENTRES[1]— 1964, 1971–1974

Table E.2

England and Wales

Year	Total live births	Number of children who attended during the year				Number of sessions held by				Total number of sessions
		Born in year of attendance	Born in previous year	Born in previous 2–5 years	Total	Medical Officers[2]	Health Visitors	GPs employed on a sessional basis	Hospital Medical Staff	
1964 ...	875,972	653,521	574,950	628,650	1,857,121	202,614	67,198	61,896	1,266	332,974
1971 ...	783,155	646,370	579,280	690,962	1,916,612	185,502	95,176	75,594	1,337	357,609
1972 ...	725,440	585,320	561,391	636,606	1,783,317	187,800	98,606	73,020	1,374	360,800
1973 ...	675,953	552,780	535,429	646,359	1,734,568	192,497	102,777	72,230	1,528	369,032
1974 ...	639,868	618,525	539,642	614,841	1,773,008	185,976	97,875	66,829	3,109	353,789

Source: DHSS
Welsh Office

[1]Includes clinics provided by voluntary organisations on behalf of local authorities.
[2]Includes sessions held jointly between medical officers and midwives.

129

VACCINATION AND IMMUNISATION

**Percentage of children born in 1969, 1970 and 1971 and vaccinated by end of 1971, 1972 and 1973 respectively
By Regional Hospital Board**

Table E.3

England and Wales

Regional Hospital Board	Whooping cough			Diphtheria			Poliomyelitis			Tetanus			Measles		
Year born	1969	1970	1971	1969	1970	1971	1969	1970	1971	1969	1970	1971	1969	1970	1971
Vaccinated by end of	1971	1972	1973	1971	1972	1973	1971	1972	1973	1971	1972	1973	1971	1972	1973
England and Wales	78	78	78	79	81	81	80	80	80	71	81	81	46	51	53
England	78	79	79	80	81	81	80	80	80	80	81	81	47	52	54
Newcastle	78	79	76	80	81	77	78	79	77	80	81	77	44	50	53
Leeds	74	78	79	75	79	80	75	79	80	75	79	80	49	56	60
Sheffield	81	80	79	82	81	80	81	80	80	82	80	80	51	56	57
East Anglian	83	81	78	85	81	79	84	81	78	84	81	79	40	48	56
NW Metropolitan	79	79	77	82	82	81	81	82	80	82	82	81	52	56	57
NE Metropolitan	84	85	86	86	87	88	86	86	88	86	87	88	49	54	56
SE Metropolitan	75	82	84	77	84	86	82	86	89	77	84	87	45	49	54
SW Metropolitan	81	80	79	83	83	82	83	82	80	83	83	82	50	53	54
Wessex	85	84	82	88	89	89	87	87	88	88	90	89	66	70	71
Oxford	85	85	84	86	86	86	85	86	86	86	86	85	67	73	70
South Western	86	85	85	87	86	86	87	85	86	88	86	86	54	62	64
Birmingham	75	75	77	80	81	83	78	78	80	80	81	83	37	43	48
Manchester	72	71	72	74	73	74	72	72	73	74	73	74	38	44	44
Liverpool	62	63	65	63	64	67	62	63	65	63	64	67	28	34	33
Wales	77	75	75	78	77	77	78	77	77	78	77	77	32	31	36

Source: DHSS
Welsh Office

NUMBERS OF CHILDREN CONSULTING GENERAL MEDICAL PRACTITIONERS AND CONSULTATION RATES FOR VACCINATION AND IMMUNISATION—1970-71

Table E.4

England and Wales

	Males			Females			All children		
	0-4	5-14	0-14	0-4	5-14	0-14	0-4	5-14	0-14
Number of patients consulting for any reason	10,113	15,822	25,935	9,257	14,944	24,201	19,370	30,766	50,136
Rate per 1,000 population	909·0	636·5	720·8	883·7	641·6	716·7	896·8	639·0	718·8
Number of consultations for any reason	42,128	47,770	89,898	36,316	45,052	81,368	78,444	92,822	171,266
Rate per 1,000 population	3,786·7	1,921·7	2,498·4	3,467·0	1,934·4	2,409·8	3,631·7	1,927·9	2,455·5
Number of consultations for vaccination and immunisation	4,453	1,514	5,967	4,251	1,244	5,495	8,704	2,758	11,462
Rate per 1,000 population	400·3	60·9	165·8	405·8	53·4	162·7	403·0	57·3	164·3
Consultation rates per 1,000 population:—									
Tuberculosis (BCG)	1·5	0·7	0·9	1·7	0·3	0·7	1·6	0·5	0·8
Smallpox	71·2	9·6	28·6	71·8	9·4	28·7	71·5	9·5	28·7
Whooping cough, Diphtheria, Tetanus	162·3	13·9	59·8	162·7	12·2	58·8	162·5	13·0	59·3
Tetanus alone	1·7	7·3	5·6	0·8	3·0	2·3	1·3	5·2	4·0
Poliomyelitis	120·5	8·2	42·9	123·4	8·6	44·2	121·9	8·4	43·5
Rubella	0·1	—	—	0·1	5·8	4·1	0·1	2·8	2·0
Measles	34·7	1·1	11·4	37·9	1·3	12·7	36·3	1·2	12·0
Typhoid, Paratyphoid	2·9	5·5	4·7	2·2	4·3	3·6	2·6	4·9	4·2
Cholera	4·9	8·0	7·0	4·9	5·2	5·1	4·9	6·7	6·1
Other diseases	0·5	6·8	4·8	0·4	3·4	2·5	0·4	3·2	3·7

Source: OPCS
Morbidity Statistics from General Practice
Second National Study 1970-1971

131

CONSULTATIONS WITH A GENERAL MEDICAL PRACTITIONER (NHS ONLY)—1971–1973

Rates per 1,000 population; Percentage distribution: by site of consultation and by age group

Table E.5   England and Wales

Site of consultation	Rate per 1,000 population			Percentage distribution		
	Age group			Age group		
	All ages	0–4	5–14	All ages	0–4	5–14

a. Persons consulting (self-reported) in a two-week reference period by site of consultation

Site of consultation	All ages	0–4	5–14	All ages	0–4	5–14
All sites[1,2]	117	149	71	104	106	104
At home	21	37	12	19	26	17
Surgery	89	99	54	80	71	79
Telephone	5	12	5	5	8	7
All persons[2]	112	140	68	100	100	100
Number of persons consulting	10,147	1,053	1,049			

b. Average number of self-reported consultations per person per year by site of consultation

Site of consultation	All ages	0–4	5–14	All ages	0–4	5–14
All sites	3·7	4·4	2·1	100	100	100
At home	0·8	1·1	0·4	21	26	17
Surgery	2·7	2·9	1·6	75	66	75
Telephone	0·2	0·3	0·1	4	7	7
Number of consultations	12,723	1,265	1,244			
Rates of surgery to at home consultations	3·6	2·5	4·3			

Source: OPCS
General Household Survey

[1]The rates per 1,000 population for "all sites" are greater than those for "all persons" (and, similarly, the percentages are greater than 100) because some respondents consulted at more than one site during the two-week reference period.

[2]The " all sites " and " all persons " figures include a very small number of respondents who consulted at other sites such as workplace or school.

CHILDREN CONSULTING GENERAL MEDICAL PRACTITIONERS
by sex, age group and Standard Region
Average number of consultations per person per year—1971–1972 combined

Table E.6   England and Wales

Standard Region	Total			Males			Females		
	All ages	0–4	5–14	All ages	0–4	5–14	All ages	0–4	5–14
England and Wales	3·7	4·6	2·1	3·2	4·5	2·2	4·3	4·7	2·0
North	4·0	4·9	1·7	3·5	5·3	1·9	4·4	4·5	1·4
Yorkshire and Humberside ...	4·2	5·5	2·3	4·0	5·3	2·3	4·3	5·7	2·4
North West ...	3·9	4·8	1·8	3·1	4·3	1·8	4·6	5·2	1·8
East Midlands ...	3·6	5·6	2·2	3·1	6·9	2·1	4·1	4·2	2·3
West Midlands...	3·3	3·6	1·5	2·8	3·1	1·9	3·7	4·3	1·2
East Anglia ...	3·6	4·1	1·8	3·1	4·3	1·6	4·1	3·8	2·1
South East ...	3·6	4·5	2·4	2·9	4·2	2·6	4·3	4·7	2·3
GLC	3·9	5·2	2·7	3·1	5·1	2·8	4·6	5·3	2·7
Outer Metropolitan Area ...	3·6	4·9	2·4	2·9	4·5	2·4	4·2	5·3	2·4
Outer South East	3·2	2·6	2·1	2·5	2·3	2·6	3·8	3·0	1·6
South West ...	3·5	3·7	1·8	3·0	4·0	1·6	4·1	3·4	2·0
Wales	4·7	4·5	2·6	4·2	4·6	2·6	5·2	4·5	2·6

Source: OPCS
General Household Survey

CHILD REFERRALS FROM GENERAL MEDICAL PRACTITIONERS TO ANOTHER AGENCY 1970-1971

Table E.7

England and Wales

	All Referrals			Referrals 0-14 to:			
	0-4	5-14	Total 0-14	In-patient	Out-patient	Investi-gation	Other
NUMBER OF REFERRALS							
Total ...	2,896	5,682	8,578	744	3,576	3,349	909
Males ...	1,638	2,920	4,558	438	2,009	1,635	476
Females	1,258	2,762	4,020	306	1,567	1,714	433
RATE PER 100 POPULATION AT RISK							
Total ...	13	12	12	1	5	5	1
Males ...	15	12	13	1	6	5	1
Females	12	12	12	1	5	5	1

Source: OPCS
Morbidity Statistics from General Practice
Second National Study 1970-1971

COMMUNITY HEALTH SERVICE: PATIENTS INSPECTED AND TREATED BY THE DENTAL SERVICE—1966-1974

Table E.8

England and Wales
Thousands

	Unit	1966	1967	1968	1969	1970	1971	1972	1973	1974
Mother and child health service: Children aged under 5 years										
Patients inspected ... ... per 1,000 children under 5	Number Rate	98·8 23·7	107·7 25·8	115·5 27·8	116·0 28·2	115·6 28·8	117·9 30·2	125·1 32·7	129·9 34·8	124·5 34·7
Patients found to require treatment per 1,000 children under 5	Number Rate	63·5 15·2	67·2 16·1	70·5 17·0	69·3 16·9	67·9 16·9	70·0 17·9	72·0 18·8	73·0 19·6	67·1 18·7
Patients treated ... ... per 1,000 children under 5	Number Rate	69·3 16·6	73·2 17·5	77·4 18·6	74·5 18·1	72·9 18·2	74·2 19·0	77·2 20·2	78·0 20·9	78·5 21·9
Total attendances for treatment... per 1,000 children under 5	Number Rate	147·5 35·4	158·9 38·1	169·0 40·7	159·6 38·9	157·5 39·3	164·8 42·2	166·0 43·4	164·8 44·1	156·8 43·7
Courses of treatment completed per 1,000 children under 5	Number Rate	54·4 13·1	59·0 14·1	61·9 14·9	59·1 14·4	57·1 14·3	60·3 15·4	62·2 16·3	62·4 16·7	61·1 17·0
School Dental Service: Children in maintained schools										
Patients inspected ... ... per 1,000 children in maintained schools	Number Rate	4,139·7 556·4	4,270·6 557·4	4,353·3 552·2	4,447·4 549·0	4,577·5 550·0	4,770·9 556·8	4,962·1 568·1	5,100·6 559·4	4,950·5 538·5
Patients found to require treatment per 1,000 children in maintained schools	Number Rate	2,363·2 317·6	2,416·7 315·4	2,431·1 303·4	2,497·2 308·3	2,557·3 307·3	2,667·2 311·3	2,719·3 311·3	2,740·3 300·5	2,574·4 280·0
Patients treated ... ... per 1,000 children in maintained schools	Number Rate	1,279·5 172·0	1,287·5 168·0	1,294·3 164·2	1,312·5 162·0	1,314·3 157·9	1,384·8 161·6	1,430·6 163·8	1,437·3 157·6	1,419·1 154·4
Total attendances for treatment... per 1,000 children in maintained schools	Number Rate	3,315·3 445·6	3,361·2 438·7	3,399·7 431·2	3,474·0 428·8	3,563·4 428·2	3,759·8 438·8	3,876·1 443·7	3,892·1 426·8	3,860·6 420·0
Courses of treatment completed per 1,000 children in maintained schools	Number Rate	1,078·1 144·9	1,104·9 144·2	1,118·6 141·9	1,138·4 140·5	1,175·0 141·2	1,221·6 142·6	1,271·1 145·5	1,294·5 142·0	1,273·6 138·5

Source: Department of Education and Science
Department of Health and Social Security
Welsh Office

SCHOOL HEALTH SERVICE IN MAINTAINED SCHOOLS: MEDICAL INSPECTIONS AND TREATMENT—1964–1974

Table E.9

England and Wales
Thousands

	1964	1965	1966	1967	1968	1969	1970	1971	1972	1973	1974
Medical inspection and treatment:											
Pupils inspected in routine medical inspections[1]	1,972	1,887	1,882	1,870	1,803	1,797	1,786	1,746	1,632	1,537	1,466
Special inspections and re-inspections[2] ...	1,538	1,478	1,393	1,364	1,291	1,215	1,179	1,245	1,177	1,143	980
Defects treated or under treatment:											
Defective vision and squint ...	533	502	491	487	469	434	435	406	408	389	349
Defects of ear, nose and throat ...	128	125	117	117	110	104	102	99	95	90	81
Orthopaedic and postural defects ...	105	94	89	85	79	79	71	70	69	79	78
Child guidance treatment	46	54	57	62	64	66	69	69	75	79	..
Speech therapy	58	62	65	68	81	82	88	94	104	109	135
Minor ailments	482	312	306	334	320	313	287	282	291	287	359

[1] No child is included more than once in the figures for any one year.
[2] The same child may be included more than once in any one year.

Source: 1964–1973 Department of Education and Science
1974 DHSS
Welsh Office

CHILDREN'S DAY CARE FACILITIES

As at 31 March 1972–1975

Table E.10

	1972	1973	1974	1975
Local authority day nurseries Number on register	23·3	25·1	25·9	26·2
Local authority part-time nursery groups Number on register	2·6	4·0	5·0*	3·2

Private facilities
    Children placed and paid for by L.A.
    Total children
	2·8	6·1	6·3	6·3

Registered premises
    All day
        Number of children permitted
	23·6	25·2	26·0	27·1

Sessional care Number of children permitted	272·3	310·1	336·3	342·5

Registered persons
    All day
        Number of children permitted
	55·7	57·0	57·2	61·3

Sessional care Number of children permitted	34·3	34·8	29·8	25·6
Total number of children under 5 Special Schools in schools (January) Other full-time Other part-time	2 296 86	3 325 101	3 334 122	3 338 141

Source: DHSS
Department of Education and Science

*Figure probably inflated due to imprecise local authority recording.

CHILDREN IN CARE OF LOCAL AUTHORITIES

As at 31 March 1972–1975

Table E.11

	1972	1973	1974	1975
Total	90·6	93·2	95·9	99·1
Accommodation				
Boarded out	29·9	29·8	30·7	31·9
In community homes	29·8	31·1	33·0	34·6
Residential accommodation for handicapped children	2·3	2·5	2·7	2·7
Charge and control of parent, etc.	15·2	16·1	16·6	18·0
Others	13·3	13·8	12·9	11·9
Age				
Under age two	3·8	4·0	3·9	4·0
Reached two but not compulsory school age ...	8·3	8·6	7·8	8·3
Of compulsory school age	51·9	59·3	63·6	66·9
Over compulsory school age	26·6	21·3	20·5	19·9

Note: Figures may not add to totals due to rounding.

Source: DHSS

CIRCUMSTANCES IN WHICH CHILDREN CAME INTO THE CARE OF LOCAL AUTHORITIES

(EXCLUDING REMAND AND INTERIM ORDERS)—1972–1975

Table E.12

England and Wales
Thousands

Reasons for children coming into care (whether or not still in care) under Section 1 of the Children Act 1948, or care orders. In cases where more than one sub-heading could apply, entry should be made under the first appropriate sub-heading	Year ending 31 March			
	1972	1973	1974	1975
Total	53·4	53·6	52·7	51·6
(a) parent dead, no guardian	0·3	0·3	0·4	0·4
(b) abandoned or lost	0·8	1·0	1·0	1·2
(c) death of mother (father not living with family, or unable to care for children)	0·7	0·7	0·7	0·6
(d) deserted by mother (father not living with family, or unable to care for children) ...	5·0	4·8	4·5	3·7
(e) confinement	4·4	3·7	2·8	2·4
(f) short-term illness (children judged likely to return to their parent or guardian within six months of the date of being received into care)	15·6	15·5	13·8	12·7
(g) Long-term illness or incapacity	1·1	1·0	1·0	0·7
(h) child illegitimate, and mother unable to provide	2·0	2·0	1·9	1·8
(i) parent or guardian in prison, or remanded in custody	0·9	1·0	0·9	0·8
(j) family homeless, because of eviction ...	1·2	0·9	0·8	0·4
(k) family homeless, through a cause other than eviction	1·8	1·9	1·6	1·2
(l) unsatisfactory home conditions	3·5	4·4	4·7	4·9
(m) other reasons	6·2	6·7	8·0	8·7
(n) care orders or court orders	9·8	9·7	10·5	12·0

Note: Figures may not add to totals due to rounding.

Source: DHSS

NUMBERS ON HANDICAP REGISTERS—1964–1975

Per 100,000 population aged under 16

Table E.13

England and Wales

Date	General Classes of Handicap	Deaf With Speech	Deaf Without Speech	Hard of Hearing	Blind	Partially Sighted
			TOTAL			
31 December 1964	38·4	8·6	14·3	13·9	19·6	20·3
31 December 1970	52·3	11·5	13·1	15·0	17·3	22·4
31 March 1974	109·9	10·3	12·6	9·7	17·9	22·0
31 March 1975	122·5	12·2	12·6	8·8	17·8	22·6
			MALES			
31 December 1964	42·9	8·6	15·6	14·6	21·1	24·3
31 December 1970	55·1	12·5	14·3	15·7	18·6	27·8
31 March 1974	117·9	11·0	13·1	9·5	19·7	26·5
31 March 1975	138·0	12·7	13·5	9·0	19·3	27·2
			FEMALES			
31 December 1964	33·8	8·5	12·9	13·4	18·0	16·1
31 December 1970	49·2	10·4	11·8	14·4	15·9	16·6
31 March 1974	101·4	9·5	12·1	9·9	16·1	17·2
31 March 1975	113·7	11·6	11·8	8·6	16·3	17·8

Source: DHSS

140

IN-PATIENTS, NHS NON-PSYCHIATRIC HOSPITALS

Discharge rates[1] per 1,000 population by sex[2] and age groups 0–19 for the years 1960–1973

Table E.14 — England and Wales

Year	0–19	0–14	Under 1 year	1–4	5–9	10–12	13–14	15–19
MALES Discharge Rates								
1960 ...	..	76	172	74	88	51	43	..
1961 ...	..	..	..	..	..	..	..	..
1962 ...	..	77	180	75	84	50	43	..
1963 ...	..	79	198	77	83	50	44	..
1964 ...	73	81	190	80	84	52	46	50
1965 ...	73	80	190	81	83	51	46	52
1966 ...	73	81	208	79	81	53	45	51
1967 ...	75	82	211	81	82	53	46	51
1968 ...	75	83	218	85	81	54	45	52
1969 ...	78	85	231	89	81	54	48	53
1970 ...	77	84	257	89	78	52	46	52
1971 ...	78	86	264	90	81	52	46	52
1972 ...	77	84	291	87	77	51	45	52
1973 ...	77	85	301	89	78	53	45	51
Index (1964=100)								
1973 ...	106	105	159	111	93	101	96	102
Estimated Discharges								
1973 ...	594,030	504,670	107,050	138,610	161,450	63,950	33,610	89,360
FEMALES[2] Discharge Rates								
1960 ...	..	60	123	51	73	46	38	..
1961 ...	..	..	..	..	..	..	..	..
1962 ...	..	58	128	51	67	41	36	..
1963 ...	..	60	146	53	65	41	39	..
1964 ...	58	60	136	54	68	41	38	52
1965 ...	59	61	141	53	66	43	41	53
1966 ...	57	59	149	54	61	40	39	50
1967 ...	59	60	164	55	63	41	39	54
1968 ...	59	60	165	55	61	40	39	55
1969 ...	58	62	171	59	60	41	41	55
1970 ...	60	61	190	60	57	39	41	57
1971 ...	62	63	200	60	58	40	42	61
1972 ...	62	62	226	59	56	40	41	60
1973 ...	61	62	239	58	55	40	41	58
Index (1964=100)								
1973 ...	105	103	176	108	82	98	107	113
Estimated Discharges								
1973 ...	448,020	350,450	80,000	85,960	108,540	46,650	29,300	97,580

Source: DHSS
Hospital In-Patient Enquiry

[1]Age specific.
[2]The figures for females in the age groups 15–19 and 0–19 do not include maternity patients.

141

IN-PATIENTS, NHS NON-PSYCHIATRIC HOSPITALS

Average number of beds occupied daily rate[1] per 1,000 population by sex[2] and age groups 0–19 for the years 1960–1973

Table E.15

England and Wales

Year	0–19	0–14	Under 1 year	1–4	5–9	10–12	13–14	15–19
			MALES					
			Average beds daily rates					
1960	..	2·3	6·6	2·1	2·3	1·7	1·4	..
1961	..	..	..	..	..	..	..	..
1962	..	2·4	7·0	2·2	2·2	1·6	1·5	..
1963	..	2·4	7·3	2·2	2·2	1·5	1·3	..
1964	2·2	2·4	7·3	2·1	2·1	1·5	1·8	1·6
1965	2·1	2·2	6·7	2·0	2·0	1·5	1·5	1·5
1966	2·0	2·2	7·5	1·9	1·8	1·5	1·3	1·5
1967	2·0	2·1	7·5	1·8	1·8	1·3	1·5	1·5
1968	1·9	1·9	6·8	1·7	1·6	1·3	1·3	1·9
1969	1·8	1·9	6·9	1·7	1·6	1·3	1·2	1·3
1970	1·7	1·8	7·7	1·7	1·4	1·1	1·1	1·3
1971	1·6	1·7	7·3	1·4	1·3	1·0	0·9	1·3
1972	1·5	1·6	8·0	1·4	1·2	1·1	1·1	1·1
1973	1·4	1·5	7·7	1·3	1·2	0·9	0·8	1·1
			Index (1964=100)					
1973	66	65	106	63	58	62	47	68
			Average number of beds occupied daily					
1973	11,013	9,113	2,752	2,051	2,568	1,105	637	1,900
			FEMALES[2]					
			Average beds daily rates					
1960	..	1·9	5·7	1·8	1·8	1·5	1·4	..
1961	..	..	..	..	..	..	..	..
1962	..	1·9	5·7	1·8	1·6	1·5	1·3	..
1963	..	1·9	6·2	1·6	1·6	1·3	1·3	..
1964	1·7	1·8	5·9	1·5	1·5	1·2	1·5	1·6
1965	1·6	1·7	5·8	1·4	1·6	1·2	1·1	1·3
1966	1·6	1·7	6·1	1·5	1·4	1·0	1·1	1·2
1967	1·5	1·6	6·0	1·3	1·3	1·0	1·1	1·3
1968	1·4	1·4	5·9	1·2	1·1	0·9	1·0	1·1
1969	1·3	1·4	5·7	1·2	1·1	0·9	1·0	1·2
1970	1·3	1·4	6·2	1·2	1·0	0·8	1·0	1·1
1971	1·3	1·3	6·3	1·1	0·9	0·8	0·9	1·2
1972	1·3	1·2	6·4	1·0	1·0	0·7	0·8	1·4
1973	1·2	1·2	6·8	0·9	0·8	0·8	0·8	1·0
			Index (1964=100)					
1973	66	66	116	62	54	66	53	65
			Average number of beds occupied daily					
1973	8,427	6,749	2,280	1,390	1,634	868	577	1,678

Source: DHSS
Hospital In-Patient Enquiry

[1]Age specific.
[2]The figure for females in the age groups 15–19 and 0–19 do not include maternity patients.

IN-PATIENTS, NHS NON-PSYCHIATRIC HOSPITALS

Mean duration of stay (days) by sex[1] and age groups 0–19 for the years 1960–1973

Table E.16   England and Wales

Year	0–19	0–14	Under 1 year	1–4	5–9	10–12	13–14	15–19
				MALES				
			Mean duration of stay (days)					
1960	..	11·1	14·0	10·5	9·5	12·1	12·1	..
1961	..	..	..	..	..	..	..	..
1962	..	11·1	14·0	10·4	9·7	11·8	12·3	..
1963	..	10·9	13·5	10·5	9·6	11·1	11·1	..
1964	10·9	10·7	14·1	9·6	9·2	10·3	14·3	11·9
1965	10·3	10·1	13·0	9·3	8·6	10·9	12·0	11·1
1966	10·1	9·9	13·3	9·0	8·2	10·6	10·6	11·2
1967	9·6	9·4	13·0	8·1	8·1	9·0	11·7	11·0
1968	9·3	8·4	11·5	7·3	7·3	8·6	10·2	13·9
1969	8·2	8·1	11·1	6·9	7·0	8·4	9·3	9·3
1970	8·1	7·9	11·0	7·0	6·8	7·5	8·5	9·4
1971	7·4	7·1	10·1	5·9	6·0	7·2	7·5	8·9
1972	7·3	7·1	10·0	5·7	5·9	7·6	9·3	7·9
1973	6·8	6·6	9·4	5·4	5·8	6·3	6·9	7·8
			Index (1964 = 100)					
1973	62	62	67	56	63	61	48	66
				FEMALES[1]				
			Mean duration of stay (days)					
1960	..	11·8	16·8	12·5	9·1	11·7	13·3	..
1961	..	..	..	..	..	..	..	..
1962	..	11·9	16·1	12·7	8·6	13·3	12·6	..
1963	..	11·3	15·6	11·2	8·8	11·4	12·2	..
1964	10·9	10·9	15·8	10·3	8·4	10·3	14·5	11·0
1965	10·1	10·4	15·0	9·8	8·8	10·2	9·7	9·2
1966	10·0	10·2	14·9	9·9	8·5	9·0	9·8	8·8
1967	9·3	9·5	13·6	8·8	7·7	9·1	9·9	8·6
1968	8·5	8·7	13·0	8·1	6·7	8·6	8·9	7·6
1969	8·0	8·2	12·2	7·5	6·4	8·0	8·9	7·4
1970	7·9	8·0	11·9	7·3	6·3	7·5	8·7	7·1
1971	7·5	7·7	11·5	6·6	6·0	7·8	8·0	7·0
1972	7·7	7·3	10·3	6·0	6·3	6·9	7·5	8·7
1973	6·9	7·0	10·4	5·9	5·5	6·8	7·2	6·3
			Index (1964 = 100)					
1973	65	64	66	57	65	66	50	65

Source: DHSS
Hospital In-Patient Enquiry

[1]The figures for females in the age groups 15–19 and 0–19 do not include maternity patients.

IN-PATIENTS, NHS NON-PSYCHIATRIC HOSPITALS—CHILDREN UNDER 15 YEARS—1973

Percentage distribution of length of stay;
Estimated numbers by age;
Index of discharge rates (1962=100)
All causes

Table E.17

England and Wales

Age group		Duration of stay													All durations
		Days									Months			1 year and over	
		0	1	2	3	4-5	6-7	8-10	11-14	15-29	1-2	3-5	6-11		
0-4	Estimated numbers	18,750	75,520	64,990	46,040	57,290	37,700	35,620	23,550	35,980	14,990	810	220	160	411,620
	Percentage	4·56	18·35	15·79	11·18	13·92	9·16	8·65	5·72	8·74	3·64	0·20	0·05	0·04	100·0
	1962 = 100	←			174	→			86	82	←	63	→		132
5-14	Estimated numbers	10,290	69,430	87,180	74,020	81,190	44,500	29,190	17,590	19,690	9,080	820	310	200	443,490
	Percentage	2·32	15·66	19·66	16·69	18·31	10·03	6·58	3·97	4·44	2·05	0·18	0·07	0·04	100·0
	1962 = 100	←			116	→			53	50	←	43	→		95
0-14	Estimated numbers	29,040	144,950	152,170	120,060	138,480	82,200	64,810	41,140	55,670	24,070	1,630	530	360	855,110
	Percentage	3·40	16·95	17·80	14·04	16·19	9·61	7·58	4·81	6·51	2·82	0·19	0·06	0·04	100·0
	1962 = 100	←			136	→			66	65	←	52	→		108

Source: DHSS
Hospital In-Patient Enquiry

IN-PATIENTS, NHS NON-PSYCHIATRIC HOSPITALS

Estimated Numbers, Percentages and Discharge Rates per 10,000 population—1973 by department, sex and age groups 0–14 years

Table E.18   England and Wales

Department	Estimated numbers of discharges		Percentage of group total		Discharge rates per 10,000 population	
	0–4	5–14	0–4	5–14	0–4	5–14
	MALES					
All departments	259,320	258,020	100·0	100·0	1,352·7	639·1
General medicine ...	3,350	4,370	1·3	1·7	17·5	10·8
Paediatrics	100,460	43,830	38·7	17·0	524·0	108·6
Infectious diseases ...	11,910	3,620	4·6	1·4	62·1	9·0
General surgery	36,500	72,780	14·1	28·3	190·4	180·3
Ear, nose and throat ...	13,560	63,050	5·2	24·4	70·7	156·2
Traumatic and orthopaedic	12,710	36,170	4·9	14·0	66·3	89·6
Ophthalmology	7,730	10,880	3·0	4·2	40·3	26·9
Plastic surgery	4,020	4,290	1·6	1·7	21·0	10·6
Special care babies ...	57,630	·	22·2	·	300·6	·
General practice units ...	2,100	2,410	0·8	0·9	11·0	6·0
Other departments ...	9,350	16,620	3·6	6·4	48·8	41·2
	FEMALES					
All departments	177,010	183,530	100·0	100·0	975·4	478·9
General medicine ...	2,640	4,430	1·5	2·4	14·5	11·6
Paediatrics	69,090	31,230	39·0	17·0	380·4	81·5
Infectious diseases ...	8,910	2,760	5·0	1·5	49·1	7·2
General surgery	11,830	37,710	6·7	20·6	65·2	98·4
Ear, nose and throat ...	9,040	56,900	5·1	31·0	49·8	148·5
Traumatic and orthopaedic	10,890	21,420	6·2	11·7	60·0	55·9
Ophthalmology ...	6,810	8,570	3·9	4·7	37·5	22·4
Plastic surgery	2,310	3,920	1·3	2·1	12·7	10·2
Special care babies ...	48,610	·	27·5	·	267·6	·
General practice units ...	1,140	1,330	0·6	0·7	6·3	3·5
Other departments ...	5,740	15,260	3·2	8·3	32·3	39·8

Source: DHSS
Hospital In-Patient Enquiry

IN-PATIENTS, NHS NON-PSYCHIATRIC HOSPITALS

Discharge rates per 10,000 population by Regional Hospital Board of residence by sex and age groups 0–14 for 1973: comparison with 1960

Table E.19 .... England and Wales

Regional Hospital Board		Discharge rates per 10,000 population				Index (1960=100)	
		1960		1973		1973	
		0–4	5–14	0–4	5–14	0–4	5–14
England and Wales... ...	M	943	665	1,285	642	136	97
	F	663	567	914	481	138	85
Newcastle	M	920	580	1,270	587	138	101
	F	701	535	974	453	139	85
Leeds	M	961	646	1,344	651	140	101
	F	648	554	1,044	505	161	91
Sheffield	M	704	543	967	551	137	101
	F	540	481	681	386	126	80
East Anglian	M	633	544	1,300	577	205	106
	F	414	438	903	475	218	108
NW Metropolitan ...	M	1,058	678	1,366	661	129	98
	F	688	586	993	503	144	86
NE Metropolitan ...	M	1,212	770	1,391	704	115	91
	F	777	672	992	529	128	79
SE Metropolitan ...	M	960	772	1,421	728	148	94
	F	641	634	979	514	153	81
SW Metropolitan ...	M	1,041	691	1,401	672	135	97
	F	681	578	1,016	538	149	93
Wessex	M	829	645	1,168	622	141	96
	F	599	564	814	450	136	80
Oxford	M	843	657	1,185	663	141	101
	F	649	577	761	463	117	80
South Western	M	802	636	1,157	631	144	99
	F	625	546	806	463	129	85
Birmingham	M	853	624	1,177	548	138	88
	F	598	524	781	425	131	81
Manchester	M	1,040	731	1,247	727	120	99
	F	735	627	905	547	123	87
Liverpool	M	1,108	723	1,525	628	138	87
	F	831	553	1,092	470	131	85
Welsh	M	971	667	1,478	696	152	104
	F	691	554	1,090	517	158	93

Source: DHSS
Hospital In-Patient Enquiry

PAEDIATRIC DEPARTMENTS

by Regional Health Authority and average number of available beds—1975

Table E.20

Regional Health Authority	Average number of available beds						Regional totals	
	Less than 10	10–24	25–49	50–74	75–99	100 and over	Number of hospitals	Number of beds
England ...	79	125	94	21	5	1	325	7,295
Northern ...	2	4	8	6	—	—	20	709
Yorkshire...	7	11	7	2	1	—	28	640
Trent ...	7	10	8	1	—	—	26	497
East Anglian	8	4	2	—	—	—	14	173
NW Thames	3	14	6	—	—	—	23	464
NE Thames	9	15	5	1	—	—	30	513
SE Thames	10	10	9	—	—	—	29	528
SW Thames	5	10	5	1	—	—	21	383
Wessex ...	6	4	7	—	—	—	17	345
Oxford ...	1	11	4	—	—	—	16	296
S Western ...	9	7	6	1	1	—	24	468
W Midlands	7	13	6	5	—	—	31	751
Mersey ...	1	3	8	2	—	1	15	582
N Western	4	8	12	2	1	—	27	720
London Post-Graduate B.G.s ...	—	1	1	—	2	—	4	226
Wales	7	12	4	4	—	—	27	550

Source: DHSS
Welsh Office

INFECTIOUS DISEASES DEPARTMENTS

by Regional Health Authority and average number of available beds—1975

Table E.21   England and Wales

Regional Health Authority	Average number of available beds						Regional totals	
	Less than 10	10–24	25–49	50–74	75–99	100 and over	Number of hospitals	Number of beds
England ...	43	50	13	7	5	2	120	2,574
Northern ...	3	1	1	1	—	—	6	152
Yorkshire ...	3	4	—	2	—	1	10	321
Trent ...	3	4	1	—	1	—	9	189
East Anglian	2	5	—	—	—	—	7	96
NW Thames	2	5	3	1	—	—	11	251
NE Thames	3	2	1	1	2	—	9	313
SE Thames	5	3	3	1	—	—	12	224
SW Thames	3	3	1	—	—	—	7	85
Wessex ...	6	2	1	—	—	—	9	105
Oxford ...	1	3	—	—	—	—	4	52
S Western ...	5	5	—	—	—	—	10	90
W Midlands	4	4	1	1	1	—	11	262
Mersey ...	2	2	—	—	—	1	5	173
N Western	1	7	1	—	1	—	10	261
London Post-Graduate B.G.s ...	—	—	—	—	—	—	—	—
Wales	4	5	3	—	—	—	12	184

Source: DHSS
Welsh Office

SPECIAL CARE BABY UNITS[1]

Average daily number of available beds and average duration of stay during the year—1964, 1971–1975

Table E.22 (a)

England and Wales

Regional Health Authority	Average number of available beds[2]						Average duration of stay in days of patients discharged or died during the year					
	1964	1971	1972	1973	1974	1975	1964	1971	1972	1973	1974	1975
England	2,317	3,610	3,731	3,873	3,932	3,978	13·3	9·8	9·5	9·3	9·1	8·8
Northern	223	331	336	334	344	333	9·7	8·8	9·0	8·5	8·3	8·1
Yorkshire	142	251	256	266	330	336	14·6	10·1	10·0	9·0	8·6	8·1
Trent	200	338	341	367	347	349	14·6	11·2	11·4	10·7	10·0	9·2
East Anglian	59	147	152	152	155	154	14·0	6·8	6·1	6·0	6·3	6·8
NW Thames	210	318	344	365	288	287	16·1	11·1	10·2	10·1	9·9	9·4
NE Thames	144	235	238	280	348	362	14·6	9·9	9·3	9·0	9·2	9·5
SE Thames	129	254	258	257	268	294	15·6	9·3	9·7	9·4	9·3	9·1
SW Thames	174	245	266	271	209	214	12·2	9·8	9·2	9·4	9·3	8·4
Wessex	84	130	138	140	194	199	10·8	8·3	8·2	8·8	9·4	8·3
Oxford	103	187	194	199	211	210	10·2	7·3	6·5	7·0	7·2	7·5
South Western	161	214	211	210	190	190	14·9	10·7	10·4	10·8	10·9	10·8
West Midlands	239	396	397	406	405	406	17·8	11·1	11·0	10·4	9·5	9·5
Mersey	175	209	221	228	246	247	11·6	8·8	8·5	8·3	8·6	8·4
North Western	275	355	379	398	377	377	13·2	11·3	10·8	11·2	11·4	10·0
London Post-Graduate B.G.s	—	—	—	—	20	20	—	—	—	—	6·8	8·9
Wales	197	238	244	237	234	232	13·8	10·6	10·2	8·9	8·1	8·0

[1] A unit under the control of a consultant paediatrician and with staff specially allocated to it.
[2] Includes unoccupied beds as well as staffed beds which are occupied.
[3] Figures for the years prior to 1974 relate to Regional Hospital Boards including teaching hospitals.

Source: DHSS
Welsh Office

149

SPECIAL CARE BABY UNITS[1]

by Regional Health Authority and average number of available beds—1975

Table E.22 (b)

England and Wales

Regional Health Authority	Average number of available beds			Regional totals	
	Less than 10	10–24	25–49	Number of hospitals	Number of beds
England	53	168	33	254	3,978
Northern	5	15	2	22	333
Yorkshire	6	13	4	23	336
Trent	4	10	5	19	349
East Anglian	3	8	—	11	154
NW Thames	2	16	1	19	287
NE Thames	5	19	1	25	362
SE Thames	8	15	1	24	294
SW Thames	3	11	1	15	214
Wessex	3	7	3	13	199
Oxford	1	7	3	11	210
South Western	3	6	2	11	190
West Midlands	5	10	7	22	406
Mersey	3	11	2	16	247
North Western	2	19	1	22	377
London Post-Graduate B.G.s	—	1	—	1	20
Wales	4	11	1	16	232

Source: DHSS
Welsh Office

A unit under the control of a consultant paediatrician and with staff specially allocated to it.

DISCHARGES FROM TWO REGIONAL CENTRES WITH NATIONAL COMPARISONS

Analysis by diagnostic group—1974

Table E.23

ICD Code	Diagnostic group	Percentage of child spells			
		Newcastle AHA(T)[1]	Durham Hospital Group[1]	Hospital for Sick Children, Gt Ormond Street[2]	England and Wales[3]
000–139	Infective and parasitic diseases ...	2·0	3·9	1·7	5·0
140–209	Malignant neoplasms	} 2·4	} 1·1	4·2	0·6
210–239	Benign and unspecified neoplasms			3·0	0·6
240–279	Endocrine, nutritional and meta-bolic diseases	1·9	2·4	7·2	2·0
280–289	Diseases of the blood	1·2	1·7	5·4	1·3
290–315	Mental disorders	0·9	1·2	3·6	0·5
320–358	Diseases of the nervous system ...	2·0	1·1	7·0	1·4
360–389	Diseases of the sense organs ...	14·3	6·8	3·4	8·0
390–459	Diseases of the circulatory system	0·5	0·5	0·8	0·3
460–519	Diseases of the respiratory system	13·9	7·4	10·0	21·1
520–577	Diseases of the digestive system...	9·0	8·5	6·5	8·5
580–629	Genito-urinary diseases	3·5	6·8	3·4	4·3
630–678	Conditions of pregnancy ...	0·8	1·9	—	0·1
680–709	Diseases of the skin	3·0	5·5	2·2	1·8
710–739	Diseases of the musculoskeletal system	1·9	2·6	1·5	1·6
740–759	Congenital anomalies	15·0	3·3	34·6	7·3
760–779	Causes of perinatal morbidity ...	0·4	2·1	1·5	8·1
780–796	Symptoms and ill-defined con-ditions	8·2	14·8	2·6	10·3
800–999	Trauma	16·3	27·0	1·4	16·5
Y40–Y79	Other conditions	2·8	1·5	—	0·4
	Total	100·0	100·0	100·0	100·0
	All child spells	13,415	1,914	7,751	855,120

Source: DHSS

1. Discharges and deaths of persons aged 16 years or less in 1974.
2. All discharges and deaths in 1974.
3. Estimated discharges and deaths in 1973 of persons aged 14 years or less.

151

PAEDIATRIC DEPARTMENTS

Day case attendances and out-patients

Table E.24

a. Totals—1954, 1964–1975

England and Wales

Paediatric Departments	1954	1964	1965	1966	1967	1968	1969	1970	1971	1972	1973	1974	1975
Day Case attendances	..								..	11,632	11,212	14,013	14,952
Out-patients—													
Annual number of clinic sessions	29,599	37,291	38,410	39,828	40,374	41,813	42,941	49,736	52,788	59,090	63,122	68,088	69,864
New out-patients[a] during the year	130,511	149,192	147,501	150,425	154,219	153,114	153,340	175,694	181,015	189,354	189,341	198,792	182,562
Total attendances per new out-patient	3·8	4·2	4·5	4·6	4·6	4·8	4·9	5·0	5·1	5·2	5·4	5·4	5·8
Total attendances during the year[a]	494,390	631,969	656,598	686,345	714,828	734,644	748,755	868,807	916,741	983,984	1,027,685	1,082,695	1,065,067

b. By Regional Hospital Board—1964, 1972 and 1973

Paediatric Departments

Regional Hospital Board	Day Case attendances[1]		Out-patients											
			Annual number of clinic sessions			New out-patients[a] during the year			Total attendances per new out-patient			Total attendances during the year[a]		
	1972	1973	1964	1972	1973	1964	1972	1973	1964	1972	1973	1964	1972	1973
Newcastle	455	346	3,666	5,475	5,717	11,475	13,718	12,896	3·3	4·6	5·1	37,817	63,257	65,549
Leeds	535	110	2,201	3,405	4,184	7,266	10,174	9,075	4·5	6·1	6·7	32,332	61,122	61,210
Sheffield	566	354	2,052	3,780	4,314	9,261	13,984	14,746	4·4	5·8	6·3	40,818	81,322	92,225
East Anglian	9	19	799	1,304	1,408	2,522	3,275	3,715	4·9	5·2	5·0	12,238	17,003	18,504
NW Metropolitan	329	990	4,396	7,157	7,033	15,287	22,764	20,006	4·4	5·5	5·7	67,751	124,919	114,625
NE Metropolitan	89	49	3,270	3,792	3,833	13,157	12,382	12,582	4·0	5·1	5·1	53,004	63,676	64,398
SE Metropolitan	96	999	2,792	5,074	5,219	11,488	16,729	16,818	3·6	4·6	4·8	41,639	76,412	80,634
SW Metropolitan	251	595	3,015	4,178	4,796	13,502	14,039	14,671	3·6	4·7	4·8	48,028	66,442	71,059
Wessex	195	1,311	990	1,940	2,301	3,161	5,021	6,457	4·2	5·7	5·6	13,337	28,679	35,918
Oxford	331	271	1,663	2,673	2,729	5,841	6,510	6,788	5·4	6·0	5·9	31,417	38,944	40,384
South Western	4,706	1,565	1,694	3,265	3,412	6,842	9,258	9,343	3·1	5·2	5·5	21,503	47,903	51,343
Birmingham	121	621	3,057	5,091	5,697	14,419	18,579	18,444	4·8	5·8	6·1	69,062	106,925	112,767
Manchester	3,397	3,298	3,503	5,564	5,621	17,357	20,532	21,273	5·3	5·0	5·1	91,065	102,442	108,732
Liverpool	475	500	1,618	2,782	2,871	4,686	9,140	9,435	4·2	4·5	4·7	19,523	41,111	43,908
Welsh	77	184	2,575	3,610	3,987	12,928	13,249	13,092	4·1	4·8	5·1	52,435	63,827	66,429

c. **By Regional Health Authority—1974 and 1975**

Paediatric Departments

Regional Health Authority	Day Case Attendances[1]		Out-patients						Total attendances during the year[3]	
			Annual number of clinic sessions		New out-patients[2] during the year		Total attendances per new out-patient			
	1974	1975	1974	1975	1974	1975	1974	1975	1974	1975
Northern	899	892	6,105	6,395	13,680	13,190	5·3	5·7	72,090	74,991
Yorkshire	358	426	5,209	4,934	13,036	10,043	5·8	7·6	75,463	76,012
Trent	618	997	3,909	4,208	12,646	13,097	6·5	6·2	82,552	80,977
East Anglian	56	121	2,012	2,101	5,388	5,229	4·7	5·0	25,405	26,352
NW Thames	1,643	2,126	4,299	4,306	12,053	10,889	5·9	6·1	70,491	66,574
NE Thames	194	237	5,169	5,279	16,862	15,099	5·3	5·8	89,109	87,242
SE Thames	838	920	5,993	6,094	19,113	17,857	4·8	5·0	91,671	88,953
SW Thames	1,871	2,920	3,772	3,879	11,654	10,334	4·5	5·1	52,806	53,208
Wessex	580	628	2,999	3,019	7,681	6,780	5·7	6·4	43,980	43,215
Oxford	371	377	2,941	2,815	7,251	5,882	6·0	6·6	43,733	38,848
South Western	1,614	1,212	3,253	3,425	8,733	8,353	5·8	5·4	50,368	44,885
West Midlands	924	1,145	6,047	6,055	19,873	18,662	6·1	6·4	121,429	119,588
Mersey	319	320	3,609	3,931	11,216	10,600	4·7	5·1	52,417	54,206
North Western	3,277	2,068	5,891	6,475	20,523	18,921	5·2	5·7	105,939	107,263
Preserved Boards of Governors hospitals	224	253	2,480	2,580	5,496	5,423	6·0	5·9	33,081	32,043
Wales	227	310	4,400	4,368	13,587	12,203	5·3	5·8	72,161	70,710

Source: DHSS
Welsh Office

Notes:
[1] Figures only available since 1972. Day cases are persons attending as non-resident patients for investigation, therapeutic test, operative procedure, or other treatment who require some form of preparation and/or period of recovery involving the provision of accommodation and services.
[2] A person whose first attendance of a continuous series at the out-patient's department for the same ailment falls within the year under review. A series is only terminated by discharge or death.
[3] Includes all attendances by patients during the year whether or not the first attendance occurred during that year.

153

ATTENDANCE AT HOSPITAL OUT-PATIENT DEPARTMENTS[1]

in a 3-month reference period—1971–1973

Table E.25

	All ages	Age group	
		0–4	5–14
Persons attending in the reference period (Rate per 1,000 population)	100	79	79
Average number of attendances per out-patient in the reference period ...	2·5	1·9	1·9
Average number of attendances per person per year	1·0	0·6	0·6
Number of persons attending	9,041	593	1,218

Source: OPCS
General Household Survey

[1]Attendance at consultative out-patients, accident and emergency departments and ancillary departments but excluding attendances at ante- or post-natal clinics.

CHARACTERISTICS OF ACCIDENT AND EMERGENCY DEPARTMENTS AND OUT-PATIENTS DEPARTMENTS USED BY CHILDREN

As at 16 April 1975

Table E.26   England and Wales

	Departments used by Hospitals with children's wards		Departments used by Hospitals with segregated children's beds in adults' wards	
	Accident and Emergency Department	Out-patients Department	Accident and Emergency Department	Out-patients Department
Percentage of departments with wholly separate facilities for children	11	27	6	18
Percentage of departments with shared facilities for adults and children	89	73	94	82
Percentage of departments which have shared facilities for adults and children having:				
(i) Separate waiting areas of facilities exclusively for children and parents ...	3	19	—	26
(ii) Specified times when children attend	—	63	—	71
Percentage of departments having a qualified RSCN nurse present when children attend for treatment or consultation:				
(i) All the time	4	8	2	9
(ii) More than half the time ...	5	4	1	1
(iii) Less than half the time ...	8	11	9	9
(iv) None of the time... ...	83	77	88	81

Source: DHSS
Welsh Office

1. Some departments are used by hospitals having both children's wards and adults' wards with segregated children's beds and therefore occur under both headings.

ACCIDENT AND EMERGENCY DEPARTMENT, FRENCHAY HOSPITAL, BRISTOL, AVON AHA
Attendance by children aged 1 to 19
March to September 1974
Table E.27

Primary diagnosis	Age group			All children 1 to 19
	1 to 4	5 to 16	17 to 19	
Brought in dead	1	2	—	3
No primary diagnosis	12	28	5	45
No abnormality	26	51	12	89
NON-TRAUMATIC				
Dental	—	5	2	7
Eye	9	16	6	31
Ear—Nose—Throat	21	40	8	69
Medical				
General medicine (including dermatology)	57	79	34	170
Psychiatric	—	7	2	9
Poisoning—overdose	95	29	17	141
Surgical				
Soft tissue-infection of hand ...	16	43	14	73
Soft tissue-infection of foot ...	6	25	21	52
Soft tissue-infections elsewhere ...	11	29	6	46
Others	7	20	8	35
Gynaecological	1	1	2	4
Orthopaedic (musculo-skeletal) ...	11	58	15	84
TRAUMATIC				
Burns and scalds	70	55	23	148
Eye	13	21	9	43
Soft tissue injuries				
Lacerations	449	1,085	225	1,759
Contusions	160	910	214	1,284
Abrasions	21	85	24	130
Bites	40	167	19	226
Foreign bodies	37	86	12	135
Head Injuries				
No loss of consciousness	283	338	34	655
Loss of consciousness	24	83	23	130
Foreign body in orifice	32	32	3	67
Musculo-skeletal injuries				
Fractured facial bones	5	22	14	41
Spinal injuries	2	16	4	22
Fractured ribs, sternum, larynx ...	—	8	3	11
Fractured pelvis	—	2	1	3
Upper limbs—fractures, dislocations, sprains	106	713	98	917
Lower limbs—fractures, dislocations, sprains	55	363	120	538
Others	3	12	2	17
Internal injury of chest, abdomen and pelvis	2	2	3	7
Peripheral nerve injuries	—	—	—	—
Vascular injuries	—	1	—	1
Tendon injuries	1	2	2	5
Total	1,576	4,436	985	6,997

Source: Avon AHA

Children under one year and also a few unable to give their age are not included in the above figures.

The total of 6,997 represents 43·9% of the 15,930 persons attending during the seven month period. The annual total for new cases seen during 1974 was 25,488.

ACCIDENT AND EMERGENCY DEPARTMENT, NOTTINGHAM CHILDREN'S HOSPITAL, NOTTINGHAMSHIRE AHA

Discharges and deaths from all accidents of children aged under 15
Year ending 31 March 1974

Table E.28

ICD No. 8th Revision	Nature of injury		All ages	Children under 5 years					Age groups	
				Under 1	1	2	3	4	Under 5	5–14
800–929	Fractures, wounds, disloca- tions, sprains, lacerations and superficial injuries ...	M F T	548 296 844	37 31 68	40 24 64	37 21 58	46 21 67	49 25 74	209 122 331	339 174 513
930–932	Foreign body in eyes or ears	M F T	4 — 4	— —	— —	2 — 2	1 — 1	— —	3 — 3	1 — 1
933–939	Foreign body in other orifices	M F T	10 7 17	2 1 3	2 1 3	2 — 2	— 2 2	— —	6 4 10	4 3 7
940	Burns to eyes	M F T	— — —	— — —	— — —	— — —	— — —	— — —	— — —	— — —
941–942	Burns confined to face, head, neck and trunk	M F T	5 6 11	— 2 2	3 1 4	— —	1 1 2	— —	4 4 8	1 2 3
943–945	Burns confined to limbs ...	M F T	5 8 13	2 2 4	— 1 1	— —	— —	— —	2 3 5	3 5 8
946–948	Burns involving head and trunk	M F T	8 — 8	2 — 2	4 — 4	— —	1 — 1	— —	7 — 7	1 — 1
949	Other burns	M F T	9 4 13	— — —	3 3 6	1 — 1	1 — 1	2 1 3	7 4 11	2 — 2
950–959	Injuries to nerves	M F T	1 — 1	— —	— —	— —	— —	— —	— — —	1 — 1
960–979	Adverse effects of medicinal agents	M F T	103 95 198	3 4 7	19 23 42	45 37 82	23 18 41	7 7 14	97 89 186	6 6 12
980–985	Toxic effects of non-medical substances	M F T	51 28 79	3 3 6	18 11 29	11 4 15	8 4 12	5 1 6	45 23 68	6 5 11
986–987	Gas poisoning	M F T	3 2 5	— 1 1	1 — 1	1 — 1	— —	— —	2 1 3	1 1 2
988–999	All other toxic and adverse effects	M F T	71 65 136	4 5 9	14 15 29	10 11 21	8 5 13	5 3 8	41 39 80	30 26 56
800–999	All accidents	M F T	818 511 1,329	53 49 102	104 79 183	109 73 182	89 51 140	68 37 105	423 289 712	395 222 617

Source: Nottinghamshire AHA

ACCIDENT AND EMERGENCY DEPARTMENT, MAYDAY HOSPITAL, CROYDON AHA

Attendance by children aged under 19

Year ending 31 December 1974

Table E.29

ICD No. 8th Revision	Diagnosis	Age group			All children under 19 years
		Under 5	5–16	17–19	
800–929	Fractures, wounds, dislocations, sprains, lacerations and superficial injuries	3,428	11,134	2,942	17,504
930–932	Foreign body in eyes or ears ...	130	129	57	316
933–939	Foreign body in other orifices ...	198	89	16	303
940	Burns to eyes	3	5	2	10
941–942	Burns confined to face, head, neck and trunk	34	30	8	72
943–945	Burns confined to limbs	109	94	41	244
946–948	Burns involving head and trunk ...	13	8	2	23
949	Other burns	31	28	10	69
950–959	Injuries to nerves	6	30	44	80
960–979	Adverse effects of medicinal agents...	170	145	136	451
980–985	Toxic effects of non-medicinal substances	53	25	16	94
986–987	Gas poisoning	6	10	3	19
988–999	All other toxic and adverse effects ...	304	948	297	1,549
800–999	All accidents	4,485	12,675	3,574	20,734
780–796*	Symptoms and ill-defined conditions	336	502	272	1,110
001–779*	All other non-accidents	788	1,258	635	2,681
001–999	All causes	5,609	14,435	4,481	24,525

Source: Croydon AHA

*These figures include medical cases referred by GPs for possible admission.

First attendance by children under 15
Year ending 31 December 1973

Table E.30

ICD No. 8th Revision	Diagnosis	Age group				All children under 15 years
		Under 5 years		5–14 years		
		New OP	Follow-up[1]	New OP	Follow-up[1]	
001–007, 009–136	Infective and parasitic diseases ...	33	9	259	8	309
008, 009	Enteritis and other diarrhoeal diseases (see Note 6)	8	1	2	1	12
140–209	Malignant neoplasms	—	1	1	2	4
210–228	Benign neoplasms	17	—	26	—	43
240–279	Endocrine, nutritional and metabolic diseases	12	2	6	4	24
280–289	Diseases of blood and blood-forming organs	3	—	8	6	17
290–315	Mental disorders	18	—	80	3	101
320–358	Diseases of the nervous system ...	2	2	15	2	21
360–379	,, ,, ,, eye (see Note 7) ...	153	2	91	4	250
380–389	,, ,, ,, ear	66	8	181	—	255
390–458	,, ,, ,, circulatory system ...	4	1	11	1	17
460–466	Acute respiratory infections (except influenza)	16	22	32	5	75
480–486	Pneumonia	—	9	1	7	17
490–493 502–519	Other diseases of the respiratory system	34	17	172	11	234
500	Hypertrophy of tonsils and adenoids	61	—	198	—	259
520–577	Diseases of the digestive system ...	71	11	92	77	251
580–629	,, ,, genito-urinary system ...	58	17	48	17	140
680–709	,, ,, the skin and sub-cutaneous tissue ...	80	9	152	7	248
710–738	Diseases of the musculo-skeletal system and connective tissue ...	51	4	111	8	174
740–759	Congenital anomalies	71	11	85	—	167
760–779	Certain causes of perinatal morbidity and mortality	4	217	—	1	222
780–796	Symptoms and ill-defined conditions	106	22	317	46	491
—	No diagnosis available	3	1	4	1	9
011–796	All non-accidents	871	366	1,892	211	3,340
800–929	Fractures, wounds, dislocations, sprains, lacerations and superficial injuries	116	65	559	212	952
930–999	All other accidents	6	15	50	5	76
001–999	All causes	993	446	2,501	428	4,368

[1] See Note 2 on page 164.

Source: Trent RHA

Table E.30 (*contd.*)

Hospital Activity Analysis: Chesterfield Royal Hospital,
Out-patient Department.

Subject: *Numbers of children attending the Chesterfield Out-patient Department for the first time in 1973.*

Notes: 1. An "Out-patient department" attendance refers to children who are referred direct to the department by G.P., consultant or other authority.

2. A "Follow-up" attendance refers to children who are referred as New Out-patients from the ward (eg. emergency admissions who have not previously attended as out-patients).

3. Out-patient and Follow-up *new* patients represent hospital morbidity for children (although it excludes A & E department); it does *not* represent total work load.

4. Definition of a child is one under 15 years of age.

5. The hospital catchment area is approximately 210,000 population; the number of children under 15 years of age is estimated at 50,000.

6. Some children may be referred direct to Sheffield, particularly to the Sheffield Children's Hospital, for special conditions such as spina bifida, leukaemia, etc., and to Lodge Moor Hospital for some infectious diseases—e.g. the young gastro-enteritics.

7. The general flow of new out-patients (aged under 15 years) is represented in the table opposite. Two groups of children are not included in the analysis:—

   (*a*) Children attending child guidance clinics which accounted for 158 new patients during 1973;

   (*b*) Children attending school ophthalmic clinics which accounted for 405 new patients during 1973.

8. The diagnostic groups refer to the *primary* diagnosis on final discharge or after 12 months care.

Table E.30 (*contd.*)

CHESTERFIELD OUT-PATIENTS—Flow of children under 15 years of age.

CHILDREN—*Numbers attending out-patient department for the first time in 1973.*

Out-patients

In-patients

Referred direct by:—

Emergency Admissions Follow-up at Out-patients

Specialty	No.
G.P. 2,598	

Specialty	No.
Paediatric	382

Consultant 128

Dermatology	4
Ear, nose and throat ...	12

Transfer from other hospital 24

Ophthalmology	7
Orthopaedic	67

Transfer from other Out-patient department ... 6

*General Surgery 372

Other Specialties 30

Accident and Emergency ... 660

Other 87

All emergencies referred from ward 874

Specialty	No.	
Paediatrics	193	
Dermatology	493	
Ear, nose and throat	822	
Ophthalmology ...	275	
Gynaecology ...	8	
General Surgery ...	311	
Orthopaedic Surgery	985	
Chest	144	
Psychiatry	92	
Dental Surgery ...	51	
Plastic Surgery ...	72	
General Medicine ...	48	3,494

All new Out-patients 4,368

In-patient

*Included in general surgery is the in-patient work of the "A & E" Consultant.

RESIDENT PATIENTS[1] IN MENTAL ILLNESS HOSPITALS AND UNITS—1954[2], 1963 and 1971

by age and time spent in current hospital

Table E.31

England and Wales

Time spent in current hospital Years	All ages			Under 15[3]					15–19		
							1971				
	1954	1963	1971	1954	1963	Total	Under 5	5–14	1954	1963	1971
All periods	152,197	132,895	109,749	183	358	563	33	530	956	1,237	1,082
Under 1	26,270	32,762	30,109	109	278	479	28	451	601	1,014	953
1—	10,697	10,002	8,685	17	38	38	2	36	113	133	90
2—	22,509	16,301	14,350	21	29	37	3	34	132	76	33
5—	23,459	14,513	12,335	29	7	6	—	6	75	4	4
10—	32,721	23,987	14,194	7	6	3	—	3	35	10	2
20 and over	36,541	35,330	30,076	.	.	.	.	.	.	.	.

Source: DHSS
Welsh Office

[1] In Regional Hospital Board mental illness hospitals and units only.
[2] 1954 figures are adjusted to equate to the same coverage as 1963 and 1971.
[3] Age break-down for under 5 and 5–14 not available for 1954 and 1963.

See page 164 for Table E32

CHILD PSYCHIATRY[1]—1964–1974

Hospital facilities used for the treatment of mental illness in children
Average daily number of available beds: Discharges and deaths: Waiting-lists: New out-patients: Total out-patient attendances

Table E.32

a. By Regional Hospital Board—1964 and 1971–1973

England and Wales

Regional Hospital Board	Average daily number of available beds				Discharges and deaths				Waiting-list at 31 December				New out-patients[2] during the year				Total out-patient attendances[3]			
	1964	1971	1972	1973	1964	1971	1972	1973	1964	1971	1972	1973	1964	1971	1972	1973	1964	1971	1972	1973
England and Wales	518	845	760	776	1,218	2,064	1,933	1,947	217	274	197	285	26,965	34,142	35,877	36,039	188,135	221,320	232,899	230,971
Newcastle	42	53	53	53	313	113	113	124	6	27	21	26	921	1,029	1,274	1,488	6,815	7,624	8,994	9,790
Leeds	18	55	42	41	57	187	182	184	—	—	—	—	683	939	912	914	6,870	6,096	4,925	5,047
Sheffield	21	71	58	58	44	206	169	171	—	11	1	3	2,140	2,736	2,644	2,732	15,531	17,029	15,433	17,526
East Anglian	—	1	1	1	11	10	8	12	—	—	—	—	1,215	941	1,104	1,311	10,472	4,584	5,066	6,915
NW Metropolitan	21	32	26	26	13	65	48	59	12	10	19	17	4,235	5,085	5,108	5,206	39,561	43,986	45,994	49,020
NE Metropolitan	20	11	27	28	71	66	115	105	—	—	16	18	3,899	4,384	4,359	4,392	22,258	23,122	24,748	19,484
SE Metropolitan	76	148	100	100	164	291	185	168	51	17	11	108	2,828	3,365	3,747	3,875	23,348	24,304	29,034	26,581
SW Metropolitan	39	37	45	51	88	135	128	133	39	17	23	11	1,578	3,074	4,021	3,381	9,539	18,827	19,609	16,131
Wessex	58	66	69	66	71	112	112	93	17	56	34	6	1,968	2,005	1,886	2,582	11,501	12,111	13,144	17,593
Oxford	104	91	66	66	118	205	180	210	37	61	—	—	1,192	2,010	1,693	1,633	7,447	12,796	13,940	13,699
South Western	39	61	63	71	48	114	126	148	2	9	14	12	1,805	2,301	2,393	2,352	10,778	14,135	13,136	12,780
Birmingham	16	58	62	64	42	144	140	109	3	20	5	7	1,220	1,921	1,884	1,871	5,739	11,300	11,417	11,278
Manchester	9	45	48	47	23	128	143	150	42	8	23	30	718	1,067	1,215	1,133	2,735	5,359	6,198	6,792
Liverpool	35	80	64	67	145	208	208	205	8	38	30	47	1,475	1,432	1,487	1,327	8,244	8,798	9,431	8,941
Welsh	20	37	37	37	10	80	76	76	—	—	—	—	1,088	1,853	2,150	1,842	7,297	11,249	11,830	9,394

b. By Regional Health Authority—1974

Regional Health Authority	Average daily number of available beds	Discharges and Deaths	Waiting-list at 31 December	New out-patients[1] during the year	Total out-patient attendances[2]
England and Wales	741	1,830	172	32,665	204,546
Northern	54	127	28	1,400	10,458
Yorkshire	42	153	—	1,289	5,871
Trent	56	176	10	2,792	16,972
East Anglian	6	14	—	1,891	10,300
NW Thames	30	60	9	3,407	26,639
NE Thames	28	97	15	4,852	25,440
SE Thames	38	107	3	4,330	23,726
SW Thames	38	95	16	972	8,897
Wessex	59	65	—	1,634	10,114
Oxford	66	199	19	2,026	17,475
South Western	68	143	6	616	2,570
West Midlands	64	105	1	1,587	9,611
Mersey	76	196	29	1,483	8,648
North Western	47	161	28	1,079	6,980
Preserved Boards of Governors ...	32	59	8	1,029	10,491
Wales	37	73	—	2,278	10,354

[1] These figures relate to facilities used for the psychiatric treatment of mental illness in children.
[2] Including child guidance clinics in hospitals.

Source: DHSS
Welsh Office

165

ADOLESCENT PSYCHIATRY UNITS   1972–1974

Hospital facilities used for the treatment of mental illness in adolescents

Average daily number of available beds: Discharges and deaths: Waiting-lists: New out-patients: Total out-patient attendances

Table E.33

a. by Regional Hospital Board—1972 and 1973

England and Wales

Regional Hospital Board	Average daily number of available beds		Discharges and deaths		Waiting-list at 31 December		New out-patients during the year		Total out-patient attendances	
	1972	1973	1972	1973	1972	1973	1972	1973	1972	1973
England and Wales	257	332	494	625	44	15	987	1,362	5,551	6,713
Newcastle	10	48	17	35	—	—	107	112	347	515
Leeds	44	45	119	130	7	—	44	61	115	164
Sheffield	43	43	97	99	6	2	177	69	1,093	424
East Anglian	10	10	3	7	—	—	153	124	613	556
NW Metropolitan	11	12	66	67	—	—	187	204	1,778	2,042
NE Metropolitan	—	—	—	—	—	—	—	—	—	—
SE Metropolitan	53	52	85	82	—	—	117	102	850	461
SW Metropolitan	—	—	—	—	—	—	30	22	173	122
Wessex	—	—	—	—	—	—	55	71	242	336
Oxford	—	32	—	26	—	—	—	323	—	815
South Western	12	12	24	33	6	—	—	19	—	38
Birmingham	20	19	9	40	25	13	45	162	208	947
Manchester	32	24	53	40	—	—	72	93	132	293
Liverpool	18	18	14	21	—	—	—	—	—	—
Welsh	4	17	7	45	—	—	—	—	—	—

b. by Regional Health Authority—1974

Regional Health Authority	Average daily number of available beds	Discharges and deaths	Waiting-list at 31 December	New out-patients during the year	Total out-patient attendances
England and Wales...	436	794	64	1,869	9,475
Northern	30	33	—	159	683
Yorkshire	46	128	8	18	63
Trent	47	101	8	113	576
East Anglian	10	3	—	357	2,153
NW Thames	24	79	—	—	—
NE Thames	—	—	—	166	1,332
SE Thames	20	28	—	65	223
SW Thames	50	86	15	147	740
Wessex	30	31	6	102	461
Oxford	32	33	—	213	952
South Western	18	48	—	4	8
West Midlands	26	48	14	208	1,366
Mersey	38	103	—	268	685
North Western	—	—	—	34	106
Preserved Boards of Governors	34	34	13	—	—
Wales	31	39	—	15	127

Source: DHSS
Welsh Office

NHS MENTAL ILLNESS HOSPITALS AND UNITS

All admissions by sex and age group; sex-/age-specific rates of admission 1964 and 1970–1974

Table E.34

England and Wales

Age group		All admissions						Rates per 100,000 home population					
		1964	1970	1971	1972	1973	1974	1964	1970	1971	1972	1973	1974
All ages	T	164,478	183,354	183,473	185,131	184,577	181,296	347	374	376	378	375	369
	M	66,408	74,901	75,186	75,821	75,644	73,762	288	314	317	318	316	308
	F	98,070	108,453	108,287	109,310	108,933	107,534	403	431	432	434	431	426
Under 5	T	77	142	184	182	191	172	2	4	5	5	5	5
	M	45	83	124	117	103	97	2	4	6	6	5	5
	F	32	59	60	65	88	75	2	3	3	3	5	4
5–9	T	333	716	759	793	759	735	10	18	19	19	19	18
	M	246	506	549	573	526	502	14	24	26	27	25	25
	F	87	210	210	220	233	233	5	11	11	11	12	12
10–14	T	841	1,320	1,404	1,410	1,418	1,429	25	38	38	37	37	36
	M	420	685	755	761	713	771	25	38	40	39	36	38
	F	421	635	649	649	705	658	26	37	36	35	38	34
15–19	T	6,744	7,967	8,164	8,366	8,128	7,635	182	241	243	243	237	219
	M	3,053	3,571	3,566	3,664	3,520	3,182	161	213	208	210	201	179
	F	3,691	4,396	4,598	4,702	4,608	4,453	204	270	280	283	276	262

Source: DHSS
Welsh Office

NHS MENTAL ILLNESS HOSPITALS AND UNITS

First admissions by sex and age group; sex-/age-specific rates of admission 1964 and 1970–1974

Table E.35

England and Wales

Age group		1964[1]	First admissions 1970	1971	1972	1973	1974	1964[1]	Rates per 100,000 home population 1970	1971	1972	1973	1974
All ages	T	79,570	67,724	65,895	63,838	62,292	59,985	168	138	135	130	127	122
	M	32,561	28,053	27,272	26,234	25,853	24,739	141	118	115	110	108	103
	F	47,009	39,671	38,623	37,604	36,439	35,246	193	158	154	149	144	140
Under 5 ...	T	65	101	136	132	125	110	2	3	3	3	3	3
	M	38	58	91	83	69	59	2	3	5	4	4	3
	F	27	43	45	49	56	51	1	2	2	3	3	3
5–9	T	280	488	499	509	519	509	8	12	12	12	13	13
	M	202	345	360	366	356	352	11	17	17	17	17	17
	F	78	143	139	143	163	157	5	7	7	7	8	8
10–14	T	658	897	975	907	937	976	20	26	27	24	24	25
	M	330	459	524	467	469	520	19	26	28	24	24	26
	F	328	438	451	440	468	456	20	26	25	24	25	24
15–19	T	4,374	4,314	4,532	4,455	4,234	3,916	118	130	135	130	123	113
	M	1,981	1,880	1,967	1,894	1,837	1,616	105	112	115	109	105	91
	F	2,393	2,434	2,565	2,561	2,397	2,300	132	149	156	154	143	135

[1] Not strictly comparable with later figures because of a change in the source question on order of admission.

Source: DHSS
Welsh Office

CHILDREN RESIDENT IN NHS MENTAL HANDICAP HOSPITALS AND UNITS

Estimated numbers and sex-/age-specific rates per 100,000 home population

Table E.36

a. By Regional Hospital Board area at 31 December 1963[1]

England and Wales

Regional Hospital Board	Numbers						Rates per 100,000 home population					
	0–4			5–14			0–4			5–14		
	Total	Males	Females	Total	Males	Females	Total	Males	Females	Total	Males	Females
England and Wales	486	270	216	6,511	4,022	2,489	12	14	11	96	116	76
England	466	261	205	6,206	3,840	2,366	13	14	11	97	117	76
Newcastle	54	27	27	573	340	233	20	20	21	118	136	98
Leeds	26	14	12	465	289	176	10	10	9	100	122	77
Sheffield	29	16	13	498	327	171	8	8	7	74	95	52
East Anglian	2	1	1	130	77	53	1	1	1	55	63	46
Combined Metropolitan[3]	177	98	79	2,292	1,409	883	16	18	15	126	151	100
Wessex	22	12	10	170	94	76	14	15	13	63	67	58
Oxford	17	9	8	281	193	88	11	12	11	110	147	72
South Western	36	19	17	527	330	197	16	16	15	124	151	96
Birmingham	50	34	16	522	293	229	12	16	8	72	79	65
Manchester	24	12	12	410	266	144	6	6	7	62	79	45
Liverpool	29	19	10	338	222	116	14	17	10	94	121	66
Wales	20	9	11	305	182	123	9	8	10	76	89	63

b. By Regional Health Authority area at 31 December 1974[2]

Regional Health Authority	Numbers						Rates per 100,000 home population					
	0–4			5–14			0–4			5–14		
	Total	Males	Females	Total	Males	Females	Total	Males	Females	Total	Males	Females
England and Wales	267	150	117	4,396	2,661	1,735	7	8	7	56	66	45
England	255	142	113	4,206	2,554	1,652	8	8	7	56	67	45
Northern	24	14	10	310	184	126	11	12	9	59	69	49
Yorkshire	15	8	7	296	169	127	6	6	5	51	57	45
Trent	15	8	7	401	229	172	4	5	4	54	60	47
East Anglian	5	5	—	111	70	41	4	7	—	40	49	31
Combined Thames[3]	61	41	20	1,270	786	484	7	9	4	61	74	48
Wessex	24	9	15	266	162	104	12	9	16	62	74	50
Oxford	17	6	11	267	146	121	10	7	13	71	75	67
South Western	22	11	11	315	189	126	10	10	11	66	77	54
West Midlands	25	14	11	446	266	180	6	7	6	51	59	42
Mersey	26	18	8	275	182	93	14	18	9	62	81	43
North Western	21	8	13	249	171	78	7	5	9	38	50	24
Wales	12	8	4	190	107	83	6	8	4	43	47	38

Source: DHSS
Welsh Office

[1] Census 1963 figures.
[2] Updated figures from the Census of Mentally Handicapped Patients 1970.
[3] The combined rate is quoted because the individual Metropolitan/Thames Regions have catchment areas in other Metropolitan/Thames Regions.

NHS MENTAL HANDICAP HOSPITALS AND UNITS

All admissions by sex and age groups; sex-/age-specific rates of admission 1964 and 1970–1974

Table E.37

England and Wales

Age group		All admissions						Sex-/age-specific rates per 100,000 home population					
		1964	1970	1971	1972	1973	1974	1964	1970	1971	1972	1973	1974
All ages ...	T	10,364	11,365	11,942	12,385	12,240	12,786	22	23	24	25	25	26
	M	5,826	6,392	6,475	7,017	6,847	7,192	25	27	27	29	29	30
	F	4,538	4,973	5,467	5,368	5,393	5,594	19	20	22	21	21	22
Under 5 ...	T	1,002	886	928	841	733	790	25	22	24	22	20	22
	M	582	491	500	447	415	432	28	24	25	23	22	23
	F	420	395	428	394	318	358	22	20	22	21	18	21
5–9 ...	T	1,643	2,336	2,376	2,184	2,097	2,284	48	57	58	53	52	57
	M	1,058	1,378	1,461	1,384	1,302	1,411	60	66	70	66	63	69
	F	585	958	915	800	795	873	35	48	46	40	40	45
10–14 ...	T	1,396	1,743	2,173	2,139	2,196	2,289	42	50	59	57	57	58
	M	886	1,083	1,260	1,332	1,335	1,394	52	60	67	69	68	69
	F	510	660	913	807	861	895	32	39	51	44	46	47
15–19 ...	T	1,988	1,662	1,661	1,742	1,904	2,201	54	50	50	51	56	63
	M	1,144	974	957	998	1,085	1,336	60	58	56	57	62	75
	F	844	688	704	744	819	865	47	42	43	45	49	51

Source: DHSS
Welsh Office

Section F
MANPOWER

The object of this section is to provide information about the medical, dental and nursing personnel available for the care of children. Few of those employed in the health and personal social services are solely engaged on the care of children. Nevertheless the figures in this section do attempt, where appropriate, to relate numbers of staff to numbers of children.

General Medical and Dental Practitioners

Table F.1 gives details of the number of general medical practitioners by type of practice for each year since 1965. It shows that there has been a slow but steady growth since 1967; the number of unrestricted principals, ie. those providing the full range of general medical services, has also been rising. The proportion of family doctors working single-handed is falling; nearly two-thirds of unrestricted principals now work in group practices compared with 58% in 1971, and just under half in 1965. The number of trainee doctors has been rising steadily while the number of doctors working as assistants has been falling—this has relevance for the development of child health services since paediatrics is one of the approved specialties in which doctors may work in their period of training in hospitals.

Table F.2 provides information on the number of unrestricted principals in each Regional Health Authority and shows that in 1974 for each unrestricted principal in England and Wales there was an average of 534 children aged 0–14 of whom 30 were under one year old, 137 aged 1–4 and 368 aged 5–14. There will be considerable variation by individual practice, of course, but the regional breakdown given in F.2 shows that in some parts of the country the ratio of children to doctors is much higher than this.   Generally speaking, it is the North of England and the Midlands, together with Oxford and Wessex, which have fewest doctors in relation to children. All the regions below the national ratio of 534:1 are in the South. However, it cannot be assumed that differences between regions in the average number of children per general medical practitioner necessarily reflect differences in the quality of service provided to children. It will be seen that there are differences between regions in the average total number of patients per doctor—and there will be similar differences in the proportion of patients who are elderly and who make, as a group, the heaviest demands on general medical practitioners' time. Social and environmental factors may also be more important in determining doctors' workload than small differences in the average number of patients per doctor. Nevertheless the figures in F.2 are sufficiently dispersed to suggest that there is greater availability of general medical practitioner time for children in the South of England and Wales than in the Midlands and the North.

Table F.3 provides regional data for the period 1971–74 on the number and percentage of unrestricted principals working in group practice. Here the regions defined are Standard Statistical Regions and not Regional Health Authorities. It will be noted that group practice is least popular in the South East.

Health Centres provide opportunities for general practitioners to work in close proximity to those providing other health services. As well as health visitors and nurses these often include dentists, opticians and pharmacists and, sometimes, specialist and other services for hospital out-patients. Table F.4 shows the

173

rapid growth in recent years in the number of health centres and the number of places available in them for general practitioners. In 1975 there were places for about 16% of all family doctors, compared with 7% in 1971 and just over 1% in 1966.

F.5 shows the growth in the number of general dental practitioners since 1964 and regional distribution of them in 1974. Even allowing for differences between regions in the proportion of children in the population, the ratio of children aged 0–14 to dentists, which averages 686 children per dentist for England and Wales as a whole, shows considerable regional variation. The general pattern is that the four Thames regions, Wessex and South Western have ratios well below the national average while other regions of England and Wales have ratios well above. Whether or not children will be less accessible to dental care in these regions will depend on a number of other factors, such as the use made of the general dental services by adults, the use made of the school dental service and the state of dental disease. However it seems incontrovertible that there are fewer dentists per head of the population in the Midlands and Northern Regions of England, and in Wales, than in the South and South West of England.

Hospital Medical Staff

Tables F.6–8 give details of certain grades of hospital medical staff who specialise in the care of children. F.6 deals with paediatricians and shows the distribution by grade and region of the 1,354 staff whose contracts were in this specialty in September 1974. Table F.7 provides somewhat similar information for the much smaller number of paediatric surgeons and F.8 for the small number of specialists in mental illness for children. National figures for 1974 and 1969 are provided to illustrate the growth in these specialties. Despite the growth in provision of paediatricians from 522 whole-time equivalents in 1964 to 1,254 whole-time equivalents in 1974 there are marked regional differences in the level of provision from 24·1 per 10,000 live births in Mersey RHA to 12·2 per 10,000 births in East Anglian and 14·5 in South West Thames RHA. The differences for paediatric surgery and mental illness children are similar. It is not possible to give more meaningful figures for hospital staff working mainly or exclusively with children since most will deal with adults also.

Community Health Staff

Tables F.9–12 provide a limited amount of information about medical and dental staff working in the community health services managed by local authorities up to April 1974 but since then by Area Health Authorities.

Table F.9 gives information for the period 1966–1973 on the employment of medical staff by local health authorities up to NHS reorganisation. It will be noted that in 1973 there were 4,305 doctors in post representing 1,189 whole-time equivalent staff. The number of whole-time equivalent doctors per 100,000 children aged 0–14 had not increased appreciably between 1966 and 1973 and at 10·2 in 1973 was only slightly higher than the figure of 9·8 for 1966. However there were marked regional variations; the regions with the highest rates being South West Metropolitan (14·8) and North West Metropolitan (13·0) followed by Manchester (12·8) and North East Metropolitan (11·6) while at the other end of the scale there were East Anglia (5·5), Oxford (6·2) and Birmingham (7·1).

174

Table F.10 provides data for the period 1964–74 on the number of medical and dental staff in the School Health Service. Over the period the numbers of all grades increased by about 25% although for medical officers the numbers have fluctuated and the increase mainly occurred since 1969. During this period the number of school children aged 5–14 increased by about 16% (see Table A.4). The number of dental auxiliaries more than doubled between 1964 and 1971.

There is considerable regional variation in the ratio of schoolchildren to school and priority dentists as the following summary shows.

Table F			Children aged 5–14 per school and priority dentist 1974	Children aged 5–14 per general dental practitioner 1974
Northern				
Northern	...	...	5,404	960
Yorkshire	...	...	6,734	821
Trent	...	...	8,129	974
West Midlands	...	...	6,597	913
Mersey	...	...	6,593	818
North Western	...	...	7,194	840
Southern				
East Anglian	...	...	6,506	816
NW Thames	...	...	5,062	384
NE Thames	...	...	5,563	575
SE Thames	...	...	5,687	567
SW Thames	...	...	4,485	439
Wessex	...	...	4,201	633
Oxford	...	...	5,681	728
South Western	...	...	4,218	546

On the whole, the six most northern regions have a much lower level of provision—broadly similar in fact to that shown in Table F.5 for the ratio of children aged 5–14 to general dental practitioners, the figures for which are also shown for ease of comparison.

Nurses

The last group of tables, F.12–16, contains information on the nursing services available for children.

Table F.12 covers community nurses by grade and region for 1974 and gives some idea of the differences in present provision between regions.

Table F.13 shows changes in the number and workload of health visitors, home nurses and midwives since 1963. It will be noted that for health visitors, although the number of staff has increased by a quarter since 1967, the average case load has fallen by 28%. So far as children under five are concerned, average case load has fallen by more than 40%; the decline in the birth rate combined with the increase in health visitors accounts for this. Children under five account for a high proportion of the health visitor's case load—over 60% in 1974—but for home nurses the proportion is negligible—about 6%. Nevertheless, the average case load has trebled since 1967 at the same time as a 36% increase in home nurses. As a result, child cases have increased fivefold since 1967. There has

175

been a decline in midwives over the period 1963–74 but a higher proportion of children were delivered in hospital, rather than at home, at the end of the period. This, combined with a falling birthrate, has resulted in an increased case load for midwives in respect of hospital confinements, but a sharply reduced case load for home confinements.

Tables F.14–16 show analyses of hospital nursing staff in post in non-psychiatric hospitals in wards containing children. They are the result of a special study undertaken in April 1975 for the use of the Child Health Services Committee.

Medical Schools

Table F.17 shows the number of paediatric clinical academic staff in British medical schools by the nature of their contract.

176

GENERAL MEDICAL PRACTITIONERS
Analysis by type of practitioner at 1 October 1965–1974

Table F.1

England and Wales

Type of practitioner	1965	1966	1967	1968	1969	1970	1971	1972	1973	1974
All practitioners: Total ...	21,489	21,302	21,293	21,397	21,505	21,709	21,910	22,343	22,686	22,885
Unrestricted principals: Total	20,014	19,832	19,837	19,957	20,133	20,357	20,633	21,044	21,266	21,510
Single-handed ...	4,855	4,770	4,661	4,527	4,362	4,244	4,152	4,044	3,901	3,849
in partnership of:										
2 doctors	6,372	6,150	5,702	5,452	5,158	5,018	4,880	4,676	4,590	4,541
3 doctors	4,770	4,764	4,926	5,067	5,253	5,265	5,262	5,475	5,415	5,430
4 doctors	2,440	2,556	2,860	2,864	3,084	3,232	3,504	3,672	3,836	3,900
5 doctors	930	895	925	1,205	1,345	1,500	1,550	1,755	1,920	2,065
6 or more doctors ...	633	690	755	838	928	1,087	1,285	1,418	1,604	1,725
Other partnerships[1] ...	14	7	8	4	3	11	—	4	—	—
Restricted principals: Total	630	609	578	545	514	474	431	398	349	318
Limited lists ...	583	563	529	499	473	438	394	361	313	279
Providing maternity medical services only	47	46	49	46	41	36	37	37	36	39
Assistants	720	740	758	757	678	667	602	586	590	480
Trainees ...	125	121	120	138	180	211	244	315	481	577

Source: DHSS
Welsh Office

[1] Partnerships in which one or more doctors were members of other partnerships, or provided restricted service only.

177

NUMBERS OF CHILDREN AGED 0–14 PER GENERAL MEDICAL PRACTITIONER
by Regional Health Authority area—1974

Table F.2

England and Wales

Regional Health Authority	No. of unre- stricted principals	Number of children per GP				Overall average list size
		0-14	Under 1	1-4	5-14	
England and Wales ...	21,510	534	30	137	368	2,372
England	20,219	537	30	137	369	2,384
Northern	1,301	577	30	143	405	2,471
Yorkshire	1,515	562	31	146	385	2,422
Trent	1,833	593	33	154	406	2,527
East Anglian	766	530	32	139	360	2,282
NW Thames	1,691	449	26	114	308	2,305
NE Thames	1,731	486	28	126	332	2,354
SE Thames	1,620	497	27	126	344	2,365
SW Thames	1,323	469	26	116	327	2,288
Wessex	1,136	548	31	140	377	2,308
Oxford	927	590	33	152	404	2,411
South Western	1,469	470	27	118	325	2,170
West Midlands	2,171	587	33	154	401	2,447
Mersey	1,045	603	31	150	422	2,466
North Western	1,691	571	32	148	391	2,465
Wales	1,291	498	28	127	342	2,191

Source: DHSS
Welsh Office

1. Figures may not add exactly to totals because of rounding
2. Based on estimate of position at 1 October 1974.
3. "Per GP" columns are the numbers of children divided by the number of unrestricted principals in that region.

UNRESTRICTED PRINCIPALS IN GROUP PRACTICE BY STANDARD REGION

Numbers and percentages at 1 October 1971–1974

Table F.3   England and Wales

Standard Region	Number in group practice				Percentage in group practice			
	1971	1972	1973	1974	1971	1972	1973	1974
England and Wales	11,986	12,821	13,533	14,019	58	61	64	65
England	11,232	12,008	12,666	13,123	58	61	63	65
North	896	950	981	985	67	70	72	76
Yorkshire and Humberside ...	1,069	1,125	1,172	1,246	55	57	60	62
East Midlands ...	889	940	1,026	1,118	65	68	72	73
East Anglia ...	462	497	529	556	64	68	71	73
South East ...	4,032	4,326	4,604	4,668	53	56	59	60
South West ...	1,136	1,194	1,269	1,374	65	67	70	71
West Midlands ...	1,250	1,362	1,397	1,425	61	64	65	66
North West ...	1,498	1,614	1,688	1,751	56	59	61	64
Wales	754	813	867	896	60	64	68	69

Source: DHSS
Welsh Office

Information for earlier years is not readily available.

GROUP PRACTICE

Doctors practising in a group may be either single-handed or in partnership.
The present definition of a group (as set out in the Statement of Fees and Allowances payable to General Medical Practitioners in England and Wales) is as follows:

(a) a group must consist of not fewer than three principals (except in some rural areas where the potential number of patients will not support more than two principals), who may or may not be in partnership;

(b) all members of the group must work in close association from a common main and central surgery, even if they sometimes also work at branch surgeries; the group should be so organised as to allow regular contact between its members. In particular, where branch surgeries are used, and the Family Practitioner Committee accept that their maintenance is essential, not less than five hours spread over not less than four regular consulting sessions a week should be spent working at the common main and central surgery by each of the members if he is to qualify for payment. Where the doctors use more than one common central surgery or where the amount of time falls just short of this, it will be open to the Family Practitioner Committee to submit particulars to the Secretary of State who will advise the Committee whether, in his view, it would be reasonable to admit the claim exceptionally;

(c) a group must provide a 24-hour service to their patients and adequate off-duty and holiday relief for each member;

(d) a group must employ help to the extent of at least one full-time person (or the equivalent in part-timers) on secretarial, nursing-receptionist or medico-social work, full-time employment being taken to mean a minimum of 38 hours a week. In a rural group of two doctors a minimum of 25 hours a week would be acceptable. Wives and members of doctors' families may be counted for this purpose, provided the Family Practitioner Committee is satisfied that they are genuinely engaged on the stipulated duties. The Secretary of State is prepared to consider exceptionally cases where, because of special circumstances, the secretarial or other help falls just short of these minima. An example of the type of case in mind is where the helper works for just short of 38 hours a week, she is unable or unwilling to increase her hours to 38, and it would be unreasonable to require the doctors to employ an additional part-timer to make up the balance of the hours required.

179

HEALTH CENTRES

Number of health centres and number of places provided for general practitioners—1966–1975

Table F.4

England and Wales

	England and Wales		England		Wales	
Year	Number of health centres	Number of places for GPs	Number of health centres	Number of places for GPs	Number of health centres	Number of places for GPs
1966	41	266	34	239	7	27
1971	306	1,625	273	1,493	33	132
1972	409	2,121	365	1,950	44	171
1973	518	2,734	464	2,520	54	214
1974	632	3,311	562	3,047	70	264
1975	708	3,764	634	3,475	74	289

Source: DHSS
Welsh Office

Note: All figures relate to the position at 31 December of the respective years.

Health centres are premises provided by Health Authorities, at which facilities may be made available for the provision of all or any of the following services:—

General medical, general dental, general ophthalmic and pharmaceutical services;

Community health services;

Specialist or other services for hospital out-patients.

GENERAL DENTAL PRACTITIONERS

Analysis by Regional Health Authority

Number and status of dentist[1] and number of children aged 5–14 per dentist[2]—1974

Table F.5   England and Wales

Regional Health Authority	All dentists	Principals	Assistants	Children aged 5–14 per dentist[2]
England and Wales—1964	10,414	9,465	949	648
1969	10,659	10,177	482	695
1974	11,528	11,273	255	686
England— 1974	11,023	10,780	243	677
Northern	546	518	28	960
Yorkshire	710	692	18	821
Trent	765	733	32	974
East Anglian	337	332	5	816
NW Thames	1,351	1,329	22	384
NE Thames	996	974	22	575
SE Thames	984	961	23	567
SW Thames	985	961	24	439
Wessex	676	670	6	633
Oxford	515	508	7	728
South Western	875	846	29	546
West Midlands	955	944	11	913
Mersey	538	529	9	818
North Western	790	783	7	840
Wales	505	493	12	875

Source: Dental Estimates Board

Note: Dentists employed as both principals and assistants have been counted only as principals.

[1] As at 30 September.
[2] Relates to the home population at 30 June.

Table F. England and Wales

| Regiona | Wte per 10,000 live births | Other Training Grades[5] | | | Wte per 10,000 live births |
		Number	Wte	Wte per 10,000 population aged 0–14	
TOTAL W DUPLICAT					
England and	0·3	306	303·2	0·28	3·5
	0·4	574	569·9	0·50	7·5
	1·3	831	802·5	0·70	12·6
TOTAL W DUPLICAT					
England and	1·3	834	802·4	0·70	12·6
England ...	1·3	795	764·1	0·70	12·7
Northe	0·8	56	56·0	0·75	14·1
Yorksh	0·6	54	53·2	0·63	11·3
Trent	0·9	72	71·6	0·66	12·1
East A	0·4	18	17·3	0·43	7·3
Thames	2·1	266	245·8	0·81	14·2
	1·4	230	216·1	0·72	12·5
NW Th	2·0	71	65·4	0·86	14·5
NE Tha	1·0	64	59·1	0·70	11·9
SE Tha	1·7	64	61·6	0·77	14·0
SW Th	0·6	31	30·0	0·48	8·9
Wessex	0·8	34	33·4	0·54	9·8
Oxford	1·2	42	39·3	0·72	12·9
South V	2·1	44	39·6	0·57	10·3
West M	0·9	79	78·8	0·62	11·2
North V	1·2	75	74·1	0·77	13·6
Mersey	0·9	55	55·0	0·87	16·9
Wales ...	1·3	39	38·3	0·60	10·6

Source: DHSS

[1] Excluding
[2] Live birth
[3] As a resul
[4] Senior hos
[5] Registrars
[6] Duplicatin a region has been eliminated and staff are allocated t
Includes t
As 7, but

T | **England and Wales**

	Other Training Grades[5]		
er) hs	Number	Wte	Wte per 10,000 live births
T(D E₃	38	38·0	0·43
ᵗ	63	63·0	0·79
ᵗ	60	60·0	0·94
T(D E₁ E₂	60	60·0	0·94
	48	48·0	0·80
-	2	2·0	0·50
-	1	1·0	0·21
⸱	11	11·0	1·86
	—	—	—
ᵇ	16	16·0	0·93
₅	11	11·0	0·64
	5	5·0	1·11
	—	—	—
-	2	2·0	0·45
₅	4	4·0	1·18
-	2	2·0	0·59
-	1	1·0	0·33
	—	—	—
-	8	8·0	1·14
	1	1·0	0·18
	6	6·0	1·85
-	12	12·0	3·32

Source: DHSS

blication within a region has been

England and Wales

per 00 ation	Other Training Grades[4]		
	Number	Wte	Wte per 10,000 population
·01	22	21·6	0·01
·02	15	15·0	0·01
·04	22	18·2	0·01
·04	22	18·1	0·01
·04	22	18·1	0·01
·02	1	0·5	0·01
·03	2	2·0	0·02
·02	—	—	—
·08	2	0·7	0·01
·06	14	12·5	0·03
·05	13	11·5	0·03
·03	1	1·0	0·01
·09	6	4·5	0·04
·03	3	3·0	0·03
·03	3	3·0	0·04
·04	—	—	—
·04	1	1·0	0·01
·02	2	1·4	0·02
·06	—	—	—
·01	—	—	—
·02	—	—	—
	—	—	—

Source: DHSS

tant did not exist in 1964.
so included in the figures for 1964 and

duplication within a region has been

by Regional Health Authority and grade

Numbers, wte and wte per 10,000 population aged 0-15 at 3[...]
National figures for 1964, 1969 and 1974

Table F.8

	Senior Registrar			Vacant	All Career Grades			Consultant	
Regional Health Authority	Number	Wte	Wte per 10,000 population	Number	Number	Wte	Wte per 10,000 population	Wte per 10,000 population	Months
TOTAL WITHOUT DUPLICATION[1]									
England and Wales				10-1964	1-178	148-0	90-0-16		
1969					1-212	156-1	90-0-12		
10-1974					1-310	267-1	12-0-18		
TOTAL WITH DUPLICATION—1974									
England and Wales				10-1	1-331	265-1	11-0-18		
England				10-1	1-320	234-6	12-0-18		
Northern					11	9-6	10-0-07		
Yorkshire					44	0-21	90-0-06		
Trent				2-9	19	17-3	01-0-04		
East Anglian					16	14-5	11-0-11		
Thames: total[2]					2-158	110-1	21-0-38		
total[3]					1-179	96-2	21-0-24		
NW Thames					32	22-7	21-0-22		
NE Thames					53	00-53	10-0-22		
SE Thames				10-1	22	20-0	12-0-10		
SW Thames					25	17-5	11-0-22		
Wessex				10-1	19	19-6	10-0-22		
Oxford				10-1	18	18-4	01-0-21		
South Western				10-1	13	11-8	20-0-11		
West Midlands				10-1	28	25-9	60-0-16		
Mersey				10-1	10	0-8	90-0-07		
North Western					12	1-01	08-0-09		
Wales				10-1	11	10-2	11-0-12		

[1] Excluding locums and staff (mainly GPs) to whom paragraph [...]
[2] As a result of a change in the method of calculation the 1974 wte figures are not [...]
[3] Senior hospital medical officers and medical assistants. There were no employed [...]
senior hospital and senior hospital dental officers. These were not shown above as 1 [...]

DOCTORS IN POST WITH LOCAL HEALTH AUTHORITIES

Numbers in post and wte in clinical work 1973
Rates per 100,000 children aged 0–14—1966, 1971–1973

Table F.9

England and Wales

Regional Hospital Board	Wte persons in clinical work Rate per 100,000 population aged 0–14				1973	
	1966	1971	1972	1973	Number in post	Wte persons in clinical work
England and Wales	9·8	9·2	9·5	10·2	4,305	1,189·2
England	9·6	8·9	9·2	10·0	4,039	1,091·6
Newcastle	7·2	7·5	8·3	8·8	231	65·1
Leeds	11·7	10·8	9·3	10·8	270	83·2
Sheffield	9·2	7·7	8·1	9·2	441	105·2
East Anglian	8·0	6·0	5·7	5·5	132	23·3
NW Metropolitan	11·1	12·4	12·7	13·0	405	121·1
NE Metropolitan	11·6	11·2	10·9	11·6	316	90·2
SE Metropolitan	9·0	7·8	7·6	8·4	349	65·0
SW Metropolitan	10·7	12·6	14·6	14·8	442	103·7
Wessex	8·0	8·5	9·7	9·3	162	45·4
Oxford	7·7	6·0	6·2	6·2	107	32·3
South Western	8·9	8·1	8·0	9·6	198	69·5
Birmingham	7·2	6·3	6·3	7·1	318	91·0
Manchester	12·3	10·7	11·6	12·8	448	140·1
Liverpool	9·3	7·9	9·1	9·9	220	56·5
Wales	14·1	13·3	14·5	15·1	266	97·6

Source: DHSS

189

MEDICAL AND DENTAL STAFF IN THE SCHOOL HEALTH SERVICE—1964–1974

Wte as at 31 December

Table F.10

England and Wales

Staff	1964	1965	1966	1967	1968	1969	1970	1971	1972	1973	1974
Medical officers	983	1,037	949	931	1,035	981	1,058	1,078	1,063	1,225	..
Dental officers[1]	1,243	1,330	1,335	1,364	1,417	1,422	1,462	1,512	1,540	1,592	1,514[2]
Dental auxiliaries[1] ...	98	124	144	156	172	178	182	200	205	217	205
Dental hygienists[1] ...	16	18	17	16	16	16	17	11	13	15	12
School nurses	2,666	2,835	2,929	2,873	3,020	3,335	3,313	3,644	3,371	3,420	4,376
Nursing assistants	300	318	317	285	280	231	355	353	366	365	236

[1]Includes sessions worked in Maternity and Child Health Service.
[2]Numbers for England at 1 September 1974 plus those for Wales at 31 December 1974.

Source: 1964–1973   Department of Education and Science
        1974   DHSS
                    Welsh Office

COMMUNITY HEALTH MEDICAL STAFF

by grade and nature of contract: 30 September 1975

Table F.11

England and Wales

	Total		Full-time		Part-time 3[1]		Part-time 4[2]		Part-time 5[3]		Honorary		Occasional Sessions[5]	
	No	Wte	No	Wte	No	Wte	No	Wte	No	Wte	No	Wte	No	Wte
Total—All Grades	6,285	2,087·7	1,358	1,358·0	465	216·3	2,699	502·4	20	3·4	16	7·5	1,727	..
Senior Medical Officer (clinical)	349	322·5	298	298·0	31	18·5	17	6·0	—	—	—	—	3	..
Clinical Medical Officer ...	2,792	978·3	577	577·0	267	138·3	1,255	262·7	4	0·3	—	—	689	..
Other Medical Staff (engaged in community medicine work only)[4]	166	98·5	84	84·0	30	7·6	49	6·3	—	—	3	0·6	—	—
Other Medical Staff (engaged in clinical work only)	1,677	447·6	178	178·0	114	39·8	1,357	220·0	15	2·8	13	6·9	—	—
Other Medical Staff (mixed work)	266	240·8	221	221·0	23	12·1	21	7·4	1	0·3	—	—	—	—
Other Medical Staff (occasional sessions)[5]	1,035	0·0	—	—	—	—	—	—	—	—	—	—	1,035	..

[1]Paid at whole-time rate.
[2]Paid at sessional rate.
[3]Member of Women Doctors Retainer Scheme: HM(72)42.
[4]Relates to time spent on non-clinical duties.
[5]No wte is collected for doctors employed on an occasional session basis.

Source: DHSS

COMMUNITY HEALTH NURSING STAFF

by Regional Health Authority—as at 30 September 1974

Table F.12

England and Wales

Regional Health Authority	Administrative Grades, Supervisors, Health Visitor Tutors		Health Visitors, Tuberculosis Visitors		Home Nurses		Midwives (employed solely on the district)		School Nursing		Other State Registered and State Enrolled Nurses	
	Wte	Wte per 10,000 population	Wte	Wte per 10,000 population	Wte	Wte per 10,000 population	Wte	Wte per 10,000 population	Wte	Wte per 10,000 population	Wte	Wte per 10,000 population
England and Wales	1,769·5	0·4	7,052·4	1·4	11,682·0	2·4	3,685·9	0·7	2,139·6	0·4	1,672·9	0·3
England	1,666·0	0·4	6,626·8	1·4	10,826·7	2·3	3,387·1	0·7	2,008·3	0·4	1,539·3	0·3
Northern	112·0	0·4	464·6	1·5	815·2	2·6	216·1	0·7	200·7	0·6	80·4	0·3
Yorkshire	119·0	0·3	471·6	1·3	764·6	2·1	295·8	0·8	135·4	0·4	145·4	0·4
Trent	149·1	0·3	575·1	1·3	1,033·9	2·3	324·0	0·7	141·5	0·3	156·9	0·3
East Anglian	48·0	0·3	231·5	1·3	408·6	2·3	186·6	1·1	39·2	0·2	24·0	0·1
NW Thames	144·7	0·4	417·8	1·2	738·0	2·1	120·1	0·3	126·5	0·4	118·4	0·3
NE Thames	172·1	0·5	446·3	1·2	748·6	2·0	214·6	0·6	195·5	0·5	174·4	0·5
SE Thames	131·7	0·4	593·9	1·6	900·3	2·5	245·4	0·7	131·2	0·4	129·0	0·4
SW Thames	104·0	0·4	519·5	1·8	757·0	2·6	102·5	0·4	108·9	0·4	85·3	0·3
Wessex	82·0	0·3	428·2	1·6	585·0	2·2	250·4	1·0	64·9	0·2	59·6	0·2
Oxford	81·0	0·4	353·2	1·6	552·2	2·5	171·5	0·8	102·8	0·5	39·4	0·2
South Western	82·5	0·3	445·3	1·4	703·7	2·2	205·2	0·7	84·4	0·3	91·5	0·3
West Midlands	191·9	0·4	700·1	1·4	1,166·5	2·3	510·4	1·0	243·2	0·5	137·2	0·3
Mersey	84·0	0·3	327·8	1·3	534·5	2·1	194·2	0·8	144·9	0·6	93·5	0·4
North Western	164·0	0·4	651·9	1·6	1,118·6	2·7	350·3	0·9	289·2	0·7	204·3	0·5
Wales	103·5	0·4	425·6	1·5	855·3	3·1	298·8	1·1	131·3	0·5	133·6	0·5

Source: DHSS / Welsh Office

COMMUNITY HEALTH NURSING STAFF–HEALTH VISITORS: HOME NURSES: MIDWIVES

Staff in post: cases attended: case loads: numbers and indices (1967=100)—1963–1974

Table F.13

England and Wales

	Staff in post: Cases attended: Case Loads							Indices (1967 = 100)						
	1963	1965	1967	1969	1971	1973	1974	1963	1965	1967	1969	1971	1973	1974
HEALTH VISITORS														
Health Visitors (Wte)	5,266	5,527	5,549	5,774	6,408	6,733	7,052	95	100	100	104	115	121	127
Total Cases attended[1] (thousands)	..	..	4,599·2	4,485·5	4,520·3	4,466·3	4,411·3	..	..	100	98	98	97	96
Rate per 1,000 total population	..	..	95·0	91·9	92·6	90·8	89·7	..	..	100	97	97	96	94
Case load	..	..	867	806	726	678	625	..	..	100	93	84	78	72
Cases of children under 5 years attended (thousands)	3,643·1	3,635·5	3,643·9	3,444·4	3,320·0	2,850·9	2,773·4	100	100	100	95	91	78	76
Rate per 1,000 children under 5 years	934	884	873	838	850	764	774	107	101	100	96	97	88	89
Case load	739	694	687	619	533	433	393	108	101	100	90	78	63	57
HOME NURSES[2]														
Home Nurses (Wte)	7,620	8,151	8,572	8,962	9,762	11,022	11,682	89	95	100	105	114	129	136
Total Cases attended[1] (thousands)	842·5	852·2	867·9	1,007·9	1,102·0	2,218·3	2,291·8	97	98	100	116	127	256	264
Rate per 1,000 total population	17·9	17·8	17·9	20·6	22·6	45·1	46·6	100	99	100	115	126	252	260
Case load	111	105	101	112	113	201	196	110	104	100	111	112	199	194
Cases of children under 5 years attended (thousands)	38·5	33·4	30·8	39·9	36·5	165·0	152·6	125	108	100	130	119	536	495
Rate per 1,000 children under 5 years	9·9	8·1	7·4	9·7	9·4	44·2	42·6	134	109	100	131	127	597	576
Case load	5·1	4·1	3·6	4·5	3·7	15·0	13·1	142	114	100	125	103	417	364
MIDWIVES														
Midwives (Wte)	5,303	5,298	5,118	4,656	4,379	4,007	3,686	104	104	100	91	86	78	72
Number of cases delivered in hospitals and other institutions[3] (thousands)	178·7	263·1	313·7	376·9	448·6	482·1	457·6	57	84	100	120	143	154	146
Case load	33·7	49·7	61·3	81·0	102·5	120·3	124·2	55	81	100	132	167	196	203
Number of domiciliary confinements attended by midwives under NHS arrangements (thousands)	270·8	236·8	184·2	130·0	87·5	41·0	26·2	147	129	100	71	48	22	14
Case load	51·1	44·7	36·0	27·9	20·0	10·2	7·1	142	124	100	78	56	28	20

Source: DHSS
Welsh Office

[1] 1973: The considerable disparity with previous years is not fully understood but is attributable in part to changes in the form of statistics collected w.e.f. 1972 which may have caused the recording of cases which had previously been excluded.

[2] From 1971, includes nursing staff undergoing district nurse training.

[3] Cases discharged and attended by midwives; includes hospital confinements conducted by domiciliary midwives (26,947 in 1974).

HOSPITAL NURSING STAFF IN POST IN WARDS CONTAINING CHILDREN: NON-PSYCHIATRIC HOSPITALS

Analysis by grade and nature of contract showing number and whole-time equivalent at 16 April 1975

Table F.14   England and Wales

Grade	Nursing Staff in Children's Wards			Nursing Staff in Adult Wards with segregated Children's Beds		
	Total wte	Whole-time number	Part-time number	Total wte	Whole-time number	Part-time number
All grades—Total	14,578	11,427	5,168	5,227	4,226	1,750
Senior grades—Total	1,226	1,226	—	798	798	—
Senior Nursing Officer I and II ...	380	380	—	236	236	—
Nursing Officer I and II	846	846	—	562	562	—
Other grades—Total	13,352	10,201	5,168	4,429	3,428	1,750
Nursing Sister/Charge Nurse I and II	1,824	1,583	408	581	495	149
Staff Nurse	1,839	1,019	1,531	657	402	495
Senior Enrolled Nurse	132	105	51	85	66	26
Enrolled Nurse	1,631	1,149	689	701	515	269
Pre-registration Student Nurse ...	3,201	3,201	—	1,093	1,093	—
Post-registration Student Nurse ...	220	220	—	40	40	—
Pupil Nurse	1,841	1,697	157	384	377	9
Nursery Nurse	392	251	225	22	11	14
Nursing Auxiliary	2,272	976	2,107	866	429	788

Source: DHSS
Welsh Office

[1] Some of the staff in the senior grades are included in the figures for children's wards and for adult wards with segregated children's beds because some hospitals have both types of ward.

[2] The staff in adult wards with segregated children's beds include all staff working in those wards, whether or not they are concerned with nursing children.

HOSPITAL NURSING STAFF IN POST IN WARDS CONTAINING CHILDREN: NON-PSYCHIATRIC HOSPITALS

Analysis by grade, nature of contract and qualification in children's nursing showing number and percentage qualified at 16 April 1975

Table F.15

England and Wales

Grade	Nursing Staff in Children's Wards						Nursing Staff in Adult Wards with segregated Children's Beds					
	Total		Whole-time		Part-time		Total		Whole-time		Part-time	
	Number qualified RSCN	Qualified RSCN as % of total	Number qualified RSCN	Qualified RSCN as % of total	Number qualified RSCN	Qualified RSCN as % of total	Number qualified RSCN	Qualified RSCN as % of total	Number qualified RSCN	Qualified RSCN as % of total	Number qualified RSCN	Qualified RSCN as % of total
All Registered Nurses—Total ...	2,367	41	1,627	43	740	38	163	7	148	9	15	2
Senior Nursing Officer I and II ...	53	14	53	14	—	—	45	19	45	19	—	—
Nursing Officer I and II ...	122	14	122	14	—	—	79	14	79	14	—	—
Nursing Sister/Charge Nurse I and II	1,130	57	954	60	176	43	25	4	18	4	7	5
Staff Nurse	1,062	42	498	49	564	37	14	2	6	1	8	2
	Number trained in Paediatric Field	Number trained in Paediatric Field as % of total	Number trained in Paediatric Field	Number trained in Paediatric Field as % of total	Number trained in Paediatric Field	Number trained in Paediatric Field as % of total	Number trained in Paediatric Field	Number trained in Paediatric Field as % of total	Number trained in Paediatric Field	Number trained in Paediatric Field as % of total	Number trained in Paediatric Field	Number trained in Paediatric Field as % of total
All Enrolled Nurses—Total ...	440	22	320	26	120	16	8	1	8	1	—	—
Senior Enrolled Nurse ...	46	29	23	22	23	45	—	—	—	—	—	—
Enrolled Nurse	394	21	297	26	97	14	8	1	8	1	—	—

Notes:

1. Some of the staff in the senior grades are included in the figures for children's wards and for adult wards with segregated children's beds because some hospitals have both types of ward.
2. The staff in adult wards with segregated children's beds include all staff working in those wards whether or not they are concerned with nursing children.

Source: DHSS
Welsh Office

195

STUDENT NURSES IN POST IN WARDS CONTAINING CHILDREN'S BEDS: NON-PSYCHIATRIC HOSPITALS

Analysis by grade of student nurse and course studied showing number and percentage of whole-time staff at 16 April 1975

Table F.16   England and Wales

| Grade | Children's Wards | | | | | | Adult Wards with segregated Children's Beds | | | | | |
| | Students studying for RSCN | | Students studying for comprehensive SRN/RSCN | | Students studying for other qualification | | Students studying for RSCN | | Students studying for comprehensive SRN/RSCN | | Students studying for other qualification | |
	No.	%	No.	%	No.	%	No.	%	No.	%	No.	%
All Student Nurses—Total ...	235	7	1,323	39	1,863	54	—	—	—	—	1,133	100
Pre-registration Student Nurse ...	57	2	1,323	41	1,821	57	—	—	—	—	1,093	100
Post-registration Student Nurse ...	178	81	—	—	42	19	—	—	—	—	40	100

Source: DHSS
Welsh Office

Note:
1. The student nurses in adult wards with segregated children's beds include all staff working in those wards, whether or not they are concerned with nursing children.

NUMBER OF MEDICAL SCHOOLS, MEDICAL STUDENTS AND PAEDIATRIC ACADEMIC STAFF—1970–1973

Table F.17   Great Britain

	1970	1971	1972	1973
Medical Schools	28	28	28	28
Students				
Annual intake	2,700	2,880	3,030	3,320
Total number of undergraduates	14,630	15,430	15,920	16,640
Paediatric Academic Staff				
Total Professors/Readers	34	33	32	34
Senior Lecturers	39	48	53	60
Lecturers	61	71	74	91
Whole-time				
Professors/Readers	32	31	32	33
Senior Lecturers	28	33	37	39
Lecturers	36	26	29	43
Part-time				
Professors/Readers	1	—	—	1
Senior Lecturers	7	7	9	13
Lecturers	11	8	11	16
Honorary				
Professors/Readers	1	2	—	—
Senior Lecturers	4	8	7	8
Lecturers	14	37	34	32
Total staff per medical school[1]	4·3	4·9	5·3	6·2
Total undergraduates per member of paediatric staff[1]	123	113	108	96

Source: DHSS

[1] Excluding staff employed at the Post-Graduate Institute of Child Health.

Section G

REGIONAL AND AREA PROFILES—1974

Table G.1 sets out certain statistics for the new health authorities at both regional and area level. Although regional figures are shown elsewhere in the statistical appendix, this is the only table to provide data for the Area Health Authorities that came into being on 1 April 1974. The table shows crude differences in indicators of need for child health services—the figures on child population and mortality fall into this category—and indications of the level of provision of service for which data on hospital beds and manpower are relevant. It should be emphasised that these figures are only crude indicators of regional differences; nevertheless the fact that they show wide differences is useful as it encourages the search for explanations. The following notes are intended to draw attention to the more obvious pitfalls in interpretation.

Population and Birth Rate

The child population estimate at mid-1974 is provided for each authority in line 1 and expressed as a % of total population for males and females separately in lines 2–4. These proportions will be affected by the age structure of the female population of child-bearing age in the area. A high proportion may not necessarily reflect high fertility. It may indicate a relative lack of old people in the area.

The proportion of males aged 0–14 is higher than the proportion of females because there are more women in the population, particularly at older ages—and this is reflected to a varying extent in all the area and regional figures.

The live birth rate shown for each area in line 5 is adjusted to take account of the extent to which the area population differs in sex/age structure from the national population. For each area the Office of Population Censuses and Surveys calculates an Area Comparability Factor (ACF) which is then multiplied by the crude birth rate for the area to provide a standardised (ie., age-adjusted) rate. As a result the locally adjusted crude birth rates reveal area differences in fertility rather than differences in fertility and age structure combined. For a more detailed explanation of ACF, see Local Authority Vital Statistics for 1974 (OPCS).

Child Mortality

The six mortality rates in lines 6–11 are defined in footnotes to the table. They are discussed in section C. In the absence of reliable information on the incidence and prevalence of child illness these figures may be interpreted as indicating broad area differences in the health care needs of children.

Health Services

Lines 12–16 provide data on the provision of hospital beds per 100,000 children 0–14 in each of five relevant specialties. The figures relate to statutory areas as distinct from management areas. This difference arises because some areas have arrangements to provide hospital services for part of a neighbouring area and may, therefore, serve a bigger population than that of the statutory area. The areas affected by these arrangements are indicated by asterisks.

Moreover the presence of a teaching hospital in an area has a distorting effect on the figures, particularly for paediatric beds. Finally, the true catchment population for a hospital's services is often impossible to estimate accurately and may vary from specialty to specialty within the same hospital. Some of the differences displayed in these tables will be explicable only with the benefit of detailed local knowledge.

Family Practitioner Services

Four indicators for family practitioner services are shown in lines 17–20. The percentage of general medical practitioners working in health centres is an indicator of the extent to which family doctors have been prepared to take the advantages of this form of practice. Health centres are defined more fully in the footnotes to Table F.4.

Two indicators of the number of children per doctor are provided. The number of GPs per 10,000 aged 0–14 is a straight ratio calculated on the basis of the statutory area population. There will be slight errors in this ratio caused by the fact that family doctors may have patients from more than one area on their lists. The number of children per general medical practitioner is not shown separately but can of course be obtained from the number of GPs per 10,000 children. (For Cleveland, 14·1 GPs per 10,000 children is equivalent to one GP for every 709 children). However, the statistics in line 18, and in line 20 where similar figures are presented for general dental practitioners, have been shown in this way to illustrate the area differences in the provision of personnel—the comparison could just as easily have been prepared, and often is, on the basis of total population rather than child population. The figures in line 20 on average list size of general medical practitioners are, of course, based on total population.

Community Nurses and School Nurses

The figures for nurses in lines 21–24 refer to the whole-time equivalents, and the population figures are for statutory areas.

200

CHILD PO I SERVICE FACILITIES
by Regional
Table G.1   England and Wales

	South Western	West Midlands	Mersey	North Western	Wales
CHILD POPULATIO Total (thousands)	690·4	1,275·0	630·3	966·4	642·4
Total (% total po	22·1	24·6	25·1	23·7	23·3
Males (% all mal	23·6	25·6	26·7	25·2	24·6
Females (% all fe	20·7	23·7	23·7	22·3	22·1
LIVE BIRTH RATE	13·0	13·4	13·1	13·6	13·7
CHILD MORTALIT					
Perinatal[1] ...	19·0	22·5	23·6	23·1	21·2
Post-neonatal[2] ...	4·2	5·1	6·1	6·7	5·6
Infant[3]	14·7	16·9	18·4	19·8	17·0
1–4 years[4] ...	0·68	0·66	0·67	0·73	0·66
5–14 years[4] ...	0·26	0·29	0·27	0·34	0·31
0–14 years[4] ...	1·16	1·30	1·31	1·54	1·34
HEALTH SERVICES					
Hospital beds p by specialty Paediatrics	67	62	80	77	90
Infectious di	13	23	28	26	29
Ear, nose an	48	46	57	61	64
Special care	28	32	39	39	36
Psychiatry...	10	5	12	5	6
FAMILY PRACTITI					
Percentage of GP	24·0	12·9	11·2	14·4	21·3
Number of GPs[5]	21·3	17·0	16·6	17·5	20·1
Average GP's[5] lis	2,170	2,447	2,466	2,465	2,191
Number of GDPs	12·7	7·5	8·5	8·2	7·9
COMMUNITY NUR					
Home nurses per	10·2	9·1	8·5	11·6	13·3
Health visitors pe	6·4	5·5	5·2	6·7	6·6
Midwives per 10,	3·6	5·0	4·0	4·6	5·8
SCHOOL HEALTH S					
Nurses per 10,00(	1·8	2·8	3·3	4·4	3·0

CHILD POPULATION, LIVE BIRTH RATE (LOCALLY ADJUSTED), CHILD MORTALITY RATES AND HEALTH SERVICE FACILITIES
by Area Health Authority—1974

Table G.1 (contd.)

		Cleveland	Cumbria	Durham	Northumberland	Gateshead	Newcastle upon Tyne	North Tyneside	South Tyneside	Sunderland
						Northern RHA				
CHILD POPULATION 0–14 (mid-1974) Total (thousands)	1	154·7	108·9	143·9	61·3	53·2	64·4	49·6	41·1	74·2
Total (% total population)	2	27·3	22·9	23·5	21·4	23·9	21·7	24·1	23·9	25·4
Males (% all males)	3	28·2	24·3	24·5	22·6	25·3	23·2	25·3	25·3	26·6
Females (% all females)	4	26·4	21·5	22·7	20·3	22·6	20·3	23·0	22·7	24·3
LIVE BIRTH RATE (locally adjusted)	5	14·6	13·0	12·6	13·1	13·1	10·8	13·2	12·5	14·1
CHILD MORTALITY RATES Perinatal[1]	6	23·6	20·8	23·2	23·1	28·4	19·8	17·5	20·5	23·5
Post-neonatal[2]	7	7·2	3·4	5·8	4·4	4·2	6·3	5·3	4·9	6·5
Infant[3]	8	19·3	15·7	18·2	15·0	16·2	16·7	14·7	15·3	20·1
1–4 years[4]	9	0·49	0·77	0·61	0·61	0·98	0·46	0·67	0·10	0·74
5–14 years[4]	10	0·24	0·36	0·28	0·35	0·22	0·26	0·20	0·20	0·41
0–14 years[4]	11	1·30	1·29	1·31	1·29	1·26	1·16	1·03	0·92	1·55
HEALTH SERVICES Hospital beds per 100,000 population 0–14 by specialty Paediatrics	12	86	74	95	7	68	316	44	90	90
Infectious diseases	13	44	7	4	—	45	—	—	—	51
Ear, nose and throat	14	62	52	17	8	—	141	52	—	83
Special care babies	15	59	35	44	29	34	68	30	32	59
Psychiatry	16	9	—	—	33	—	30	—	—	—
FAMILY PRACTITIONER COUNCILS Percentage of GPs[5] in Health Centres ...	17	32·6	3·1	25·5	20·3	5·4	16·0	35·4	27·1	71·8
Number of GPs[5] per 10,000 population 0–14	18	14·1	20·6	16·1	21·7	17·3	22·4	15·9	17·0	14·8
Average GP's[5] list size	19	2,707	2,179	2,628	2,127	2,540	2,295	2,609	2,537	2,717
Number of GPs[6] per 10,000 population 0–14	20	5·5	8·4	6·0	7·8	6·4	13·0	10·3	6·1	5·4
COMMUNITY NURSES Home nurses per 10,000 population 0–14 ...	21	9·4	14·5	9·7	14·7	10·1	11·5	11·2	7·2	9·5
Health visitors per 10,000 population 0–14 ...	22	4·3	7·5	6·0	8·0	5·5	8·9	7·0	4·9	5·4
Midwives per 10,000 women 15–44	23	4·4	2·2	3·6	2·2	3·5	2·6	1·6	7·1	5·8
SCHOOL HEALTH SERVICE Nurses per 10,000 population 5–14	24	6·7	1·5	2·5	1·5	1·6	6·8	2·7	4·1	5·2

[1] Still births plus deaths of infants under one week per 1,000 live and still births.
[2] Deaths of infants aged 4 weeks and under one year per 1,000 live births.
[3] Deaths of infants under one year of age per 1,000 live births.
[4] Deaths per 1,000 population.
[5] General Medical Practitioners.
[6] General Dental Practitioners.

NOTE: It is necessary to be careful when comparing rates for AHAs as the provision of services may be changing rapidly over time.

Sources: Population statistics (item 1), live birth rates (item 5) and mortality rates (items 6–11) supplied by OPCS. Hospital services statistics (items 12–16) from DHSS Form SH3.

CHILD POPULATION, LIVE BIRTH RATE (LOCALLY ADJUSTED), CHILD MORTALITY RATES AND HEALTH SERVICE FACILITIES
by Area Health Authority—1974

Table G.1 (contd.)

		Yorkshire RHA						
		Humberside*	North Yorkshire*	Bradford*	Calderdale	Kirklees	Leeds	Wakefield
CHILD POPULATION 0–14 (mid-1974) Total (thousands)	1	210·8	143·7	113·2	45·1	91·1	171·0	75·9
Total (% total population)	2	24·9	22·2	24·6	23·4	24·3	22·8	24·9
Males (% all males)	3	25·9	23·6	26·2	24·8	25·7	24·1	25·9
Females (% all females)	4	23·8	20·8	23·0	22·2	22·9	21·7	23·9
LIVE BIRTH RATE (locally adjusted) ...	5	14·0	12·4	15·1	14·6	14·5	12·6	13·2
CHILD MORTALITY RATES Perinatal[1]	6	22·8	20·2	23·7	21·1	21·9	22·6	21·2
Post-neonatal[2]	7	6·0	6·2	11·9	5·7	6·6	8·2	6·4
Infant[3]	8	17·3	17·0	25·2	19·8	17·5	22·1	17·3
1–4 years[4]	9	0·61	0·63	0·90	1·20	0·77	0·66	0·60
–14 years[4]	10	0·21	0·30	0·48	0·32	0·21	0·31	0·21
0–14 years[4]	11	1·26	1·27	2·03	1·69	1·36	1·61	1·23
HEALTH SERVICES Hospital beds per 100,000 population 0–14 by specialty Paediatrics	12	70	54	149	55	66	60	96
Infectious diseases	13	46	17	64	—	—	91	17
Ear, nose and throat	14	49	42	49	55	52	57	68
Special care babies	15	35	28	51	40	42	35	54
Psychiatry...	16	8	8	—	—	—	9	—
FAMILY PRACTITIONER COUNCILS Percentage of GPs[5] in Health Centres ...	17	18·3	18·0	29·5	23·7	17·2	12·2	15·1
Number of GPs[5] per 10,000 population 0–14	18	17·1	20·9	16·8	16·9	16·6	18·2	16·6
Average GP's[5] list size	19	2,435	2,150	2,545	2,608	2,481	2,459	2,569
Number of GDPs[6] per 10,000 population 0–14	20	5·5	10·6	8·9	7·3	7·2	11·1	6·9
COMMUNITY NURSES Home nurses per 10,000 population 0–14 ...	21	8·9	8·7	9·0	12·0	8·6	8·8	8·9
Health visitors per 10,000 population 0–14...	22	5·4	5·8	5·7	4·5	5·4	6·3	4·3
Midwives per 10,000 women 15–44 ...	23	2·3	4·3	8·1	5·7	2·9	4·4	5·6
SHCOOL HEALTH SERVICE Nurses per 10,000 population 5–14	24	3·0	1·9	1·6	5·0	2·4	1·9	1·4

[1] Still births plus deaths of infants under one week per 1,000 live and still births.
[2] Deaths of infants aged 4 weeks and under one year per 1,000 live births.
[3] Deaths of infants under one year of age per 1,000 live births.
[4] Deaths per 1,000 population.
[5] General Medical Practitioners.
[6] General Dental Practitioners.

NOTE: It is necessary to be careful when comparing rates for AHAs as the provision of services may be changing rapidly over time.

Sources: Population statistics (item 1), live birth rates (item 5) and mortality rates (items 6–11) supplied by OPCS. Hospital services statistics (items 12–16) from DHSS Form SH3.

by Area Health Authority—1974

Table G.1 (contd.)

		Trent RHA								East Anglian RHA		
		Derbyshire*	Leicestershire	Lincolnshire	Nottinghamshire	Barnsley	Doncaster	Rotherham	Sheffield	Cambridgeshire*	Norfolk*	Suffolk*
CHILD POPULATION 0–14 (mid-1974) Total (thousands)	1	208·3	199·9	121·1	239·9	55·9	72·5	63·7	125·1	128·5	144·6	133·1
Total (% total population) ...	2	23·3	24·1	23·3	24·5	24·9	25·5	25·7	22·3	23·7	22·2	23·5
Males (% all males)	3	24·3	25·0	24·2	25·5	25·7	26·0	26·6	23·5	24·4	23·3	24·5
Females (% all females) ...	4	22·4	23·2	22·5	23·6	24·1	25·0	24·8	21·1	23·1	21·2	22·5
LIVE BIRTH RATE (locally adjusted)	5	12·9	13·0	13·7	13·4	13·2	13·6	13·9	11·5	13·2	13·6	14·0
CHILD MORTALITY RATES Perinatal[1]	6	21·2	22·5	21·5	19·6	22·4	17·8	23·5	20·5	15·9	17·2	16·7
Post-neonatal[2]	7	4·5	4·4	4·1	6·1	4·8	7·2	5·5	4·4	4·7	3·4	5·6
Infant[3]	8	15·4	16·1	13·6	15·9	16·2	16·7	14·8	17·2	13·7	12·1	16·6
1–4 years[4]	9	0·54	0·55	0·48	0·52	0·95	0·60	0·40	0·62	0·80	0·96	0·46
5–14 years[4]	10	0·29	0·29	0·31	0·28	0·34	0·28	0·16	0·35	0·32	0·23	0·25
0–14 years[4]	11	1·19	1·25	1·13	1·18	1·32	1·24	1·02	1·25	1·25	1·11	1·25
HEALTH SERVICES Hospital beds per 100,000 population 0–14 by specialty Paediatrics	12	26	27	40	45	85	41	40	97	42	38	36
Infectious diseases	13	3	15	16	10	7	28	—	66	31	25	17
Ear, nose and throat	14	36	27	53	44	47	50	52	47	37	48	31
Special care babies	15	23	23	40	40	36	34	22	40	37	51	26
Psychiatry	16	6	—	10	7	—	2	—	11	4	—	—
FAMILY PRACTITIONER COUNCILS Percentage of GPs[5] in Health Centres	17	8·5	13·8	18·3	39·4	23·9	33·3	4·7	18·6	19·2	5·6	8·0
Number of GPs[5] per 10,000 population 0–14	18	18·0	17·4	18·9	15·5	16·5	15·3	13·3	17·6	17·4	20·1	18·9
Average GP's[5] list size	19	2,474	2,421	2,251	2,656	2,577	2,745	2,718	2,653	2,361	2,212	2,292
Number of GDPs[6] per 10,000 population 0–14	20	6·7	7·8	6·8	6·6	4·8	5·2	6·0	10·2	7·2	8·5	9·2
COMMUNITY NURSES Home nurses per 10,000 population 0–14	21	8·9	9·9	9·5	7·6	9·9	9·2	8·4	14·2	9·7	12·6	7·7
Health visitors per 10,000 population 0–14	22	5·6	6·0	4·9	4·8	2·8	5·4	5·7	5·8	6·3	6·4	4·4
Midwives per 10,000 women 15–44	23	4·9	4·3	1·1	4·0	—	3·7	4·8	3·8	4·8	7·9	3·7
SCHOOL HEALTH SERVICE Nurses per 10,000 population 5–14	24	1·0	1·7	2·2	1·8	2·5	0·3	5·0	2·7	2·0	1·2	1·1

[1] Still births plus deaths of infants under one week per 1,000 live and still births.
[2] Deaths of infants aged 4 weeks and under one year per 1,000 live births.
[3] Deaths of infants under one year of age per 1,000 live births.
[4] Deaths per 1,000 population.
[5] General Medical Practitioners.
[6] General Dental Practitioners.

NOTE: It is necessary to be careful when comparing rates for AHAs as the provision of services may be changing rapidly over time.

Sources: Population statistics (item 1), live birth rates (item 5) and mortality rates (item 6–11) supplied by OPCS. Hospital services statistics (items 12–16) from DHSS Form SH3.

CHILD POPULATION, LIVE BIRTH RATE (LOCALLY ADJUSTED), CHILD MORTALITY RATES AND HEALTH SERVICE FACILITIES
by Area Health Authority—1974

Table G.1 (contd.)

		NW Thames RHA						
		Bedfordshire	Hertfordshire*	Barnet*	Brent and Harrow*	Ealing, Hammersmith and Hounslow*	Hillingdon	Kensington, Chelsea and Westminster*
CHILD POPULATION 0–14 (mid-1974) Total (thousands)	1	130·6	234·3	59·9	101·9	137·0	51·9	43·3
Total (% total population)	2	26·9	24·8	20·1	21·6	20·5	22·3	11·2
Males (% all males)	3	27·8	25·7	21·8	22·8	21·6	23·1	12·4
Females (% all females)	4	26·0	24·0	18·7	20·5	19·4	21·4	10·2
LIVE BIRTH RATE (locally adjusted)	5	14·8	12·3	11·3	12·7	12·1	12·2	6·2
CHILD MORTALITY RATES Perinatal[1]	6	19·9	15·5	16·8	19·1	19·7	15·6	13·4
Post-neonatal[2]	7	4·5	4·5	5·0	4·7	2·9	4·1	4·4
Infant[3]	8	15·2	13·8	12·6	15·3	15·0	11·7	13·0
1–4 years[4]	9	0·84	0·46	0·92	0·68	0·68	0·23	1·17
5–14 years[4]	10	0·35	0·27	0·17	0·27	0·18	0·22	0·17
0–14 years[4]	11	1·34	1·00	1·10	1·32	1·28	0·87	1·55
HEALTH SERVICES Hospital beds per 100,000 population 0–14 by specialty Paediatrics	12	10	48	73	42	84	82	276
Infectious diseases	13	3	8	37	69	54	69	53
Ear, nose and throat	14	27	32	75	35	53	66	291
Special care babies	15	36	29	54	33	40	28	83
Psychiatry...	16	—	8	—	—	8	—	2
FAMILY PRACTITIONER COUNCILS Percentage of GPs[5] in Health Centres ...	17	10·4	6·1	6·5	6·1	10·3	13·0	—
Number of GPs[5] per 10,000 population 0–14	18	14·8	17·6	25·9	24·1	24·7	17·7	58·4
Average GP's[5] list size	19	2,675	2,453	2,126	2,248	2,291	2,549	1,879
Number of GDPs[6] per 10,000 population 0–14	20	6·7	12·1	22·9	17·4	18·6	13·1	79·2
COMMUNITY NURSES Home nurses per 10,000 population 0–14 ...	21	9·3	9·5	7·7	9·4	7·1	10·7	22·7
Health visitors per 10,000 population 0–14 ...	22	4·5	3·7	5·0	6·9	6·1	7·9	11·0
Midwives per 10,000 women 15–44	23	5·2	0·6	1·0	1·1	1·4	3·4	0·7
SCHOOL HEALTH SERVICE Nurses per 10,000 population 5–14	24	2·6	1·7	1·7	1·8	3·5	0·8	6·9

[1] Still births plus deaths of infants under one week per 1,000 live and still births.
[2] Deaths of infants aged 4 weeks and under one year per 1,000 live births.
[3] Deaths of infants under one year of age per 1,000 live births.
[4] Deaths per 1,000 population.
[5] General Medical Practitioners.
[6] General Dental Practitioners.

NOTE: It is necessary to be careful when comparing rates for AHAs as the provision of services may be changing rapidly over time.

Sources: Population statistics (item 1), live birth rates (item 5) and mortality rates (items 6–11) supplied by OPCS. Hospital services statistics (items 12–16) from DHSS Form SH3.

CHILD POPULATION, LIVE BIRTH RATE (LOCALLY ADJUSTED), CHILD MORTALITY RATES AND HEALTH SERVICE FACILITIES
by Area Health Authority—1974

Table G.1 (contd.)

			NE Thames RHA				
		Essex	Barking and Havering	Camden and Islington*	City and East London	Enfield and Haringey*	Redbridge and Waltham Forest
CHILD POPULATION 0–14 (mid-1974) Total (thousands)	1	346·6	92·4	60·8	135·1	107·3	98·4
Total (% total population)	2	24·6	23·0	16·4	22·7	21·8	21·1
Males (% all males)	3	26·0	24·2	17·6	23·7	23·3	22·5
Females (% all females)...	4	23·3	21·9	15·3	21·7	20·4	19·8
LIVE BIRTH RATE (locally adjusted)	5	13·3	12·9	9·1	14·7	12·3	13·0
CHILD MORTALITY RATES Perinatal[1]	6	19·3	17·5	17·2	21·1	16·5	22·2
Post-neonatal[2]	7	5·0	4·7	4·5	5·8	6·5	4·8
Infant[3]	8	14·9	14·6	14·9	16·4	16·4	18·3
1–4 years[4]	9	0·55	0·69	0·78	0·93	0·43	0·49
5–14 years[4]	10	0·33	0·33	0·27	0·28	0·24	0·27
0–14 years[4]	11	1·19	1·21	1·46	1·49	1·25	1·44
HEALTH SERVICES Hospital beds per 100,000 population 0–14 by specialty Paediatrics	12	42	49	164	77	60	66
Infectious diseases	13	9	50	126	58	65	11
Ear, nose and throat	14	33	47	158	86	50	58
Special care babies	15	28	43	98	57	35	38
Psychiatry	16	5	—	0·5	—	—	12
FAMILY PRACTITIONER COUNCILS Percentage of GPs[5] in Health Centres	17	8·6	2·3	11·1	6·0	7·6	10·1
Number of GPs[5] per 10,000 population 0–14	18	16·5	18·6	38·7	22·1	22·0	22·1
Average GP's[5] list size	19	2,458	2,489	2,137	2,293	2,333	2,318
Number of GDPs[6] per 10,000 population 0–14 ...	20	8·2	8·5	31·1	11·9	13·6	13·9
COMMUNITY NURSES Home nurses per 10,000 population 0–14	21	6·8	8·7	17·4	8·8	7·6	12·8
Health visitors per 10,000 population 0–14	22	3·9	3·8	16·5	4·5	5·0	6·1
Midwives per 10,000 women 15–44	23	4·4	3·6	1·5	0·2	2·9	2·5
SCHOOL HEALTH SERVICE Nurses per 10,000 population 5–14	24	2·1	0·9	11·1	5·1	2·8	4·1

[1] Still births plus deaths of infants under one week per 1,000 live and still births.
[2] Deaths of infants aged 4 weeks and under one year per 1,000 live births.
[3] Deaths of infants under one year of age per 1,000 live births.
[4] Deaths per 1,000 population.
[5] General Medical Practitioners.
[6] General Dental Practitioners.

NOTE: It is necessary to be careful when comparing rates for AHAs as the provision of services may be changing rapidly over time.

Sources: Population statistics (item 1), live birth rates (item 5) and mortality rates (items 6–11) supplied by OPCS. Hospital services statistics (items 12–16) from DHSS Form SH3.

CHILD POPULATION, LIVE BIRTH RATE (LOCALLY ADJUSTED), CHILD MORTALITY RATES AND HEALTH SERVICE FACILITIES
by Area Health Authority—1974

Table G.1 (contd.)

		SE Thames RHA					SW Thames RHA				
		East Sussex	Kent	Greenwich and Bexley	Bromley	Lambeth, Southwark and Lewisham	Surrey*	West Sussex	Croydon	Kingston and Richmond*	Merton, Sutton and Wandsworth*
CHILD POPULATION 0–14 (mid-1974) Total (thousands)	1	122·4	344·7	98·2	65·7	174·0	227·3	127·7	76·6	57·8	130·7
Total (% total population)	2	18·6	23·9	22·8	21·8	22·0	22·6	20·7	23·3	18·9	20·6
Males (% all males)	3	20·9	25·6	23·9	23·4	23·5	23·9	23·0	24·7	20·2	22·2
Females (% all females)	4	16·6	22·3	21·9	20·3	20·6	21·3	18·8	22·0	17·7	19·2
LIVE BIRTH RATE (locally adjusted) ...	5	11·4	13·3	12·4	11·4	12·2	11·6	12·4	11·8	10·9	12·1
CHILD MORTALITY RATES Perinatal[1]	6	20·0	17·8	19·1	16·9	23·4	16·4	15·0	18·5	22·7	21·2
Post-neonatal[2]	7	4·1	4·3	4·4	3·2	7·1	3·4	2·8	4·5	5·5	4·3
Infant[3]	8	13·3	13·6	14·7	12·4	20·9	13·2	10·5	13·5	18·1	16·9
1–4 years[4]	9	1·01	0·43	0·56	0·30	0·82	0·51	0·58	0·76	0·34	0·57
5–14 years[4]	10	0·36	0·27	0·22	0·24	0·28	0·24	0·19	0·26	0·20	0·38
0–10 years[4]	11	1·19	1·04	1·11	0·88	1·59	0·97	0·82	1·08	1·31	1·44
HEALTH SERVICES Hospital beds per 100,000 population 0–14 by specialty Paediatrics	12	71	35	91	57	98	44	41	14	56	146
Infectious diseases	13	14	28	—	25	61	7	16	59	—	46
Ear, nose and throat	14	78	47	14	77	100	39	42	22	36	78
Special care babies	15	32	20	52	47	44	37	40	26	23	31
Psychiatry	16	8	7	—	—	2	—	0·8	—	—	29
FAMILY PRACTITIONER COUNCILS Percentage of GPs[5] in Health Centres ...	17	4·2	4·3	2·2	—	4·1	20·4	25·5	12·0	5·4	4·6
Number of GPs[5] per 10,000 population 0–14	18	25·2	17·6	18·9	19·9	22·2	19·9	21·5	18·5	25·6	23·5
Average GP's[5] list size	19	2,191	2,422	2,496	2,426	2,331	2,280	2,291	2,437	2,259	2,243
Number of GDPs[6] per 10,000 population 0–14	20	16·3	10·0	11·2	14·5	13·4	15·5	15·5	16·2	19·0	15·4
COMMUNITY NURSES Home nurses per 10,000 population 0–14	21	18·1	9·3	12·8	6·1	11·0	11·5	13·6	9·2	18·6	11·0
Health visitors per 10,000 population 0–14	22	9·7	6·5	7·3	6·7	7·9	6·5	7·8	6·6	10·4	13·1
Midwives per 10,000 women 15–44 ...	23	2·6	5·8	2·6	3·6	1·0	1·1	2·0	2·1	2·3	2·6
SCHOOL HEALTH SERVICE Nurses per 10,000 population 5–14 ...	24	2·2	0·3	5·0	1·0	5·4	1·4	0·6	4·0	1·7	5·9

[1] Still births plus deaths of infants under one week per 1,000 live and still births.
[2] Deaths of infants aged 4 weeks and under one year per 1,000 live births.
[3] Deaths of infants under one year of age per 1,000 live births.
[4] Deaths per 1,000 population.
[5] General Dental Practitioners.

NOTE: It is necessary to be careful when comparing rates of AHAs as the provision of services may be changing rapidly over time.

Sources: Population statistics (item 1), live birth rates (item 5) and mortality rates (items 6–11) supplied by OPCS. Hospital services statistics (items 12–16) from DHSS Form SH3.

CHILD POPULATION, LIVE BIRTH RATE (LOCALLY ADJUSTED), CHILD MORTALITY RATES AND HEALTH SERVICE FACILITIES
by Area Health Authority—1974

Table G.1 (contd.)

		Wessex RHA				Oxford RHA			
		Dorset	Hampshire*	Wiltshire*	Isle of Wight	Berkshire*	Buckinghamshire*	Northamptonshire	Oxfordshire*
CHILD POPULATION 0–14 (mid-1974) Total (thousands)	1	114·9	354·9	130·1	22·3	165·7	127·4	124·6	129·0
Total (% total population) ...	2	20·2	24·7	25·6	20·1	25·3	25·6	25·1	24·1
Males (% all males)	3	21·7	26·2	26·7	21·7	26·2	26·5	26·1	25·0
Females (% all females)	4	18·8	23·4	24·6	18·7	24·5	24·7	24·1	23·2
LIVE BIRTH RATE (locally adjusted)	5	11·7	13·3	14·4	12·3	13·0	13·6	14·4	11·9
CHILD MORTALITY RATES Perinatal[1]	6	18·1	18·1	16·4	20·6	16·4	15·8	17·2	13·2
Post-neonatal[2]	7	4·4	5·3	6·2	4·2	3·7	2·3	5·2	7·1
Infant[3]	8	13·0	15·5	15·1	15·0	14·1	11·5	15·0	14·3
1–4 years[4]	9	0·55	0·66	0·76	1·13	0·51	0·46	0·69	0·56
5–14 years[4]	10	0·36	0·23	0·18	0·06	0·30	0·25	0·42	0·34
0–14 years[4]	11	1·08	1·18	1·18	1·12	1·10	0·93	1·36	1·16
HEALTH SERVICES Hospital beds per 100,000 population 0–14 by specialty Paediatrics	12	85	46	67	25	82	22	58	47
Infectious diseases	13	18	18	16	19	11	—	15	9
Ear, nose and throat... ...	14	49	44	66	46	44	38	44	29
Special care babies	15	37	22	52	18	51	19	39	43
Psychiatry	16	—	10	17	—	22	—	—	23
FAMILY PRACTITIONER COUNCILS Percentage of GPs[5] in Health Centres	17	5·7	21·9	10·0	13·2	—	18·0	15·6	34·8
Number of GPs[5] per 10,000 population 0–14	18	22·7	17·2	16·2	23·8	17·4	16·2	16·0	18·1
Average GP's[5] list size	19	2,188	2,369	2,324	2,130	2,420	2,436	2,602	2,212
Number of GDPs[6] per 10,000 population 0–14	20	15·0	10·5	7·8	13·9	10·6	9·3	6·8	10·6
COMMUNITY NURSES Home nurses per 10,000 population 0–14	21	10·5	8·2	10·8	14·4	11·5	9·6	9·4	9·4
Health visitors per 10,000 population 0–14	22	7·5	5·9	9·0	7·6	9·0	5·2	5·0	5·9
Midwives per 10,000 women 15–44	23	6·6	5·2	2·9	4·6	4·8	4·3	5·0	1·3
SCHOOL HEALTH SERVICE Nurses per 10,000 population 5–14	24	0·3	1·9	1·4	3·0	4·5	2·6	2·6	0·8

[1] Still births plus deaths of infants under one week per 1,000 live and still births.
[2] Deaths of infants aged 4 weeks and under one year per 1,000 live births.
[3] Deaths of infants under one year of age per 1,000 live births.
[4] Deaths per 1,000 population.
[5] General Medical Practitioners.
[6] General Dental Practitioners.

NOTE: It is necessary to be careful when comparing rates for AHAs as the provision of services may be changing rapidly over time.

Sources: Population statistics (item 1), live birth rates (item 5) and mortality rates (items 6–11) supplied by OPCS. Hospital services statistics (items 12–16) from DHSS Form SH3.

CHILD POPULATION, LIVE BIRTH RATE (LOCALLY ADJUSTED), CHILD MORTALITY RATES AND HEALTH SERVICE FACILITIES
by Area Health Authority—1974

Table G.1 (contd.)

		South Western RHA					Mersey RHA				
		Avon*	Cornwall and Isles of Scilly	Devon	Gloucestershire	Somerset*	Cheshire*	Liverpool*	St. Helens with Knowsley	Sefton*	Wirral*
CHILD POPULATION 0–14 (mid-1974) Total (thousands)	1	207·8	86·0	190·5	116·8	89·3	227·6	129·4	110·3	76·2	86·8
Total (% total population)	2	22·7	21·5	20·5	24·1	22·3	25·2	23·1	28·5	24·8	24·7
Males (% all males)	3	24·1	23·0	22·3	25·4	23·6	26·3	24·8	30·0	26·9	26·6
Females (% all females)	4	21·4	20·2	18·9	22·8	21·1	24·0	21·5	27·1	22·9	23·1
LIVE BIRTH RATE (locally adjusted) ...	5	12·9	13·4	13·1	13·0	13·1	12·9	12·0	15·4	13·3	12·7
CHILD MORTALITY RATES Perinatal[1]	6	20·3	19·9	17·8	17·5	19·6	21·5	27·1	24·3	24·3	22·3
Post-neonatal[2]	7	4·1	3·1	3·7	5·7	4·6	5·1	6·3	6·8	7·0	6·9
Infant[3]	8	15·7	13·5	13·2	15·6	15·2	16·4	19·5	18·8	18·4	21·8
1–4 years[4]	9	0·54	0·44	0·95	0·62	0·79	0·58	0·87	0·78	0·73	0·43
5–14 years[4]	10	0·25	0·26	0·23	0·28	0·29	0·29	0·29	0·24	0·24	0·24
0–14 years[4]	11	1·18	1·06	1·15	1·17	1·24	1·20	1·45	1·37	1·25	1·37
HEALTH SERVICES Hospital beds per 100,000 population 0–14 by specialty Paediatrics	12	73	41	79	62	63	58	116	34	15	202
Infectious diseases	13	3	2	32	8	16	—	10	8	160	38
Ear, nose and throat	14	58	24	62	40	25	34	82	47	101	56
Special care babies	15	25	23	32	27	29	32	63	22	43	42
Psychiatry	16	2	—	9	8	41	—	32	—	24	19
FAMILY PRACTITIONER COUNCILS Percentage of GPs[5] in Health Centres ...	17	25·0	17·9	31·8	17·6	17·6	16·6	2·4	15·4	7·0	12·3
Number of GPs[5] per 10,000 population 0–14	18	19·2	22·8	23·8	19·9	20·9	16·1	19·4	12·3	16·9	18·7
Average GP's[5] list size	19	2,352	2,100	2,061	2,138	2,159	2,438	2,476	2,785	2,461	2,252
Number of GDPs[6] per 10,000 population 0–14	20	13·3	11·6	14·0	11·2	11·3	8·8	9·7	5·0	8·9	10·3
COMMUNITY NURSES Home Nurses per 10,000 population 0–14	21	8·3	11·5	11·4	9·5	11·7	8·0	10·9	8·6	9·0	5·6
Health visitors per 10,000 population 0–14	22	6·5	7·0	7·0	5·3	6·0	5·5	5·8	3·0	6·3	5·3
Midwives per 10,000 women 15–44 ...	23	3·3	0·2	4·7	5·2	2·9	4·2	3·1	5·3	3·3	4·0
SCHOOL HEALTH SERVICE Nurses per 10,000 population 5–14 ...	24	2·1	0·8	2·7	1·1	0·9	2·0	6·7	2·4	3·7	2·3

[1] Still births plus deaths of infants under one week per 1,000 live and still births.
[2] Deaths of infants aged 4 weeks and under one year per 1,000 live births.
[3] Deaths of infants under one year of age per 1,000 live births.
[4] Deaths per 1,000 population.
[5] General Medical Practitioners.
[6] General Dental Practitioners.

NOTE: It is necessary to be careful when comparing rates for AHAs as the provision of services may be changing rapidly over time.

Sources: Population statistics (item 1), live birth rates (item 5) and mortality rates (items 6–11) supplied by OPCS. Hospital services statistics (iterms 12–16) from DHSS Form SH3.

210

CHILD POPULATION, LIVE BIRTH RATE (LOCALLY ADJUSTED), CHILD MORTALITY RATES AND HEALTH SERVICE FACILITIES
by Area Health Authority—1974

Table G.1 (contd.)

		Hereford and Worcestershire	Salop	Staffordshire	Warwickshire	Birmingham	Coventry	Dudley	Sandwell	Solihull	Walsall	Wolverhampton
						West Midlands RHA						
CHILD POPULATION 0–14 (mid-1974) Total (thousands)	1	139·3	87·3	245·2	119·3	255·5	86·3	72·3	76·8	53·8	71·3	67·9
Total (% total population) ...	2	23·8	24·6	24·8	25·4	23·5	25·8	24·1	24·0	26·9	26·2	25·4
Males (% all males)	3	24·9	25·6	25·7	26·2	24·5	26·5	25·0	25·0	28·0	27·1	26·4
Females (% all females)	4	22·8	23·7	23·8	24·7	22·6	25·0	23·3	23·1	25·9	25·4	24·4
LIVE BIRTH RATE (locally adjusted)	5	12·9	13·2	13·1	13·1	13·3	13·3	13·7	14·3	13·1	14·1	14·8
CHILD MORTALITY RATES Perinatal[1]	6	18·5	20·1	23·8	20·9	22·6	23·2	20·6	27·0	20·1	25·9	25·9
Post-neonatal[2]	7	3·9	4·5	5·6	3·3	5·9	5·3	4·4	4·8	6·4	8·2	4·0
Infant[3]	8	13·4	14·4	17·6	13·7	18·4	18·9	15·5	18·0	16·2	22·2	17·9
1–4 years[4]	9	0·61	0·82	0·41	0·96	0·75	0·53	0·56	0·71	0·57	0·68	0
5–14 years[4]	10	0·27	0·46	0·27	0·28	0·26	0·29	0·37	0·23	0·43	0·28	0·19
0–14 years[4]	11	1·09	1·33	1·26	1·17	1·42	1·33	1·27	1·35	1·25	1·51	1·35
HEALTH SERVICES Hospital beds per 100,000 population 0–14 by specialty Paediatrics	12	49	53	40	90	94	91	40	38	—	47	92
Infectious diseases	13	27	30	22	—	41	15	25	30	—	—	18
Ear, nose and throat ...	14	28	50	39	49	67	61	45	26	—	33	66
Special care babies	15	25	25	12	36	52	35	7	18	99	19	38
Psychiatry	16	—	—	—	22	15	—	—	—	—	—	—
FAMILY PRACTITIONER COUNCILS Percentage of GPs[5] in Health Centres	17	18·4	9·6	22·8	5·1	15·6	5·0	6·2	10·8	—	13·3	—
Number of GPs[5] per 10,000 population 0–14	18	19·1	18·0	15·6	16·3	19·3	16·3	15·6	18·1	13·0	14·7	16·1
Average GP's[5] list size ...	19	2,183	2,296	2,565	2,446	2,408	2,526	2,635	2,475	2,508	2,591	2,575
Number of GDPs[6] per 10,000 population 0–14	20	9·0	8·7	6·1	7·8	9·2	7·3	5·1	7·8	7·6	4·8	6·2
COMMUNITY NURSES Home nurses per 10,000 population 0–14	21	11·5	8·4	7·9	12·7	10·3	9·3	9·4	7·7	7·8	4·5	6·4
Health visitors per 10,000 population 0–14	22	6·8	5·9	5·6	7·0	5·4	6·6	4·1	4·3	3·2	3·6	4·7
Midwives per 10,000 women 15–44	23	5·4	2·5	5·2	6·2	5·7	5·1	0·8	5·9	4·7	3·7	7·7
SCHOOL HEALTH SERVICE Nurses per 10,000 population 5–14	24	1·6	1·2	0·8	2·1	3·8	4·6	2·1	5·3	1·4	7·2	4·2

[1] Still births plus deaths of infants under one week per 1,000 live and still births.
[2] Deaths of infants aged 4 weeks and under one year per 1,000 live births.
[3] Deaths of infants under one year of age per 1,000 live births.
[4] Deaths per 1,000 population.
[5] General Medical Practitioners.
[6] General Dental Practitioners.

NOTE: It is necessary to be careful when comparing rates for AHAs as the provision of services may be changing rapidly over time.

Sources: Population statistics (item 1), live birth rates (item 5) and mortality rates (items 6–11) supplied by OPCS. Hospital services statistics (items 12–16) from DHSS Form SH3.

CHILD POPULATION, LIVE BIRTH RATE (LOCALLY ADJUSTED), CHILD MORTALITY RATES AND HEALTH SERVICE FACILITIES
by Area Health Authority—1974

Table G.1 (contd.)

		North Western RHA										
		Lancashire	Bolton	Bury	Manchester	Oldham	Rochdale	Salford	Stockport	Tameside*	Trafford	Wigan
CHILD POPULATION 0–14 (mid-1974) Total (thousands)	1	310·9	63·9	44·9	114·9	55·0	54·4	65·5	72·6	53·4	54·6	76·3
Total (% total population) ...	2	22·7	24·4	24·9	22·4	24·5	25·8	24·4	24·6	24·0	24·0	24·9
Males (% all males)	3	24·3	25·8	26·6	23·8	26·0	27·2	25·8	25·9	25·2	25·3	26·2
Females (% all females)	4	21·1	23·1	23·3	21·0	23·1	24·6	23·1	23·4	22·9	22·8	23·5
LIVE BIRTH RATE (locally adjusted)	5	14·1	13·9	13·9	12·5	14·7	15·3	13·7	13·1	13·8	12·7	14·6
CHILD MORTALITY RATES Perinatal[1]	6	22·7	22·3	22·6	23·9	23·6	24·8	24·3	21·0	29·0	24·5	19·1
Post-neonatal[2]	7	6·8	6·3	5·9	8·0	8·3	7·5	5·7	7·2	7·5	5·5	4·5
Infant[3]	8	19·6	17·3	16·2	21·4	23·3	22·8	20·0	18·6	23·3	20·4	16·0
1–4 years[4]	9	0·58	0·82	0·67	0·85	0·81	1·03	0·84	0·79	0·99	0·73	0·56
5–14 years[4]	10	0·33	0·30	0·26	0·41	0·38	0·27	0·48	0·34	0·22	0·29	0·38
0–14 years[4]	11	1·50	1·41	1·27	1·71	1·85	1·75	1·62	1·40	1·69	1·41	1·38
HEALTH SERVICES Hospital beds per 100,000 population 0–14 by specialty Paediatrics	12	60	67	40	181	60	102	99	45	54	48	61
Infectious diseases	13	32	16	—	84	—	—	—	61	—	—	—
Ear, nose and throat ...	14	49	50	25	154	34	48	56	38	28	108	42
Special care babies	15	34	54	38	72	26	28	32	30	45	33	33
Psychiatry	16	5	17	—	19	—	—	—	—	—	—	—
FAMILY PRACTITIONER COUNCILS Percentage of GPs[5] in Health Centres	17	15·7	21·4	24·6	4·4	10·0	11·4	16·7	30·0	2·4	14·4	13·6
Number of GPs[5] per 10,000 population 0–14	18	18·3	16·1	14·5	21·6	16·4	14·5	18·3	16·5	15·5	17·8	15·5
Average GP's[5] list size	19	2,437	2,576	2,675	2,223	2,516	2,707	2,360	2,446	2,673	2,413	2,717
Number of GDPs[6] per 10,000 population 0–14	20	7·9	8·0	10·2	11·1	5·8	6·8	5·8	10·1	6·7	10·6	5·9
COMMUNITY NURSES Home nurses per 10,000 population 0–14	21	13·8	9·3	11·8	10·9	11·2	9·6	11·0	7·3	11·1	11·6	11·8
Health visitors per 10,000 population 0–14	22	6·3	7·7	6·4	7·0	6·7	8·1	6·9	5·8	6·8	8·3	6·2
Midwives per 10,000 women 15–44	23	3·3	3·4	5·0	4·5	7·3	6·0	6·3	4·0	8·1	3·0	5·9
SCHOOL HEALTH SERVICE Nurses per 10,000 population 5–14	24	2·3	4·7	5·3	8·8	4·6	5·4	6·4	3·6	3·4	3·5	4·4

[1] Still births plus deaths of infants under one week per 1,000 live and still births.
[2] Deaths of infants aged 4 weeks and under one year per 1,000 live births.
[3] Deaths of infants under one year of age per 1,000 live births.
[4] Deaths per 1,000 population.
[5] General Medical Practitioners.
[6] General Dental Practitioners.

NOTE: It is necessary to be careful when comparing rates for AHAs as the provision of services may be changing rapidly over time.

Sources: Population statistics (item 1), live birth rates (item 5) and mortality rates (items 6–11) supplied by OPCS. Hospital services statistics (items 12–16) from DHSS Form SH3.

Table G.1 (contd.)

		Wales							
		Clwyd	Dyfed	Gwent	Gwynedd	Mid-Glamorgan	Powys	South Glamorgan	West Glamorgan
CHILD POPULATION 0–14 (mid-1974) Total (thousands)	1	88·9	68·0	107·3	50·4	129·2	21·4	92·8	84·4
Total (% total population) ...	2	23·9	21·3	24·4	22·6	24·0	21·3	23·7	22·7
Males (% all males)	3	25·6	22·5	25·5	24·4	25·1	21·9	24·9	24·0
Females (% all females)	4	22·2	20·2	23·3	20·9	23·0	20·7	22·5	21·5
LIVE BIRTH RATE (locally adjusted)	5	14·4	13·0	13·2	14·7	14·3	14·3	12·7	13·1
CHILD MORTALITY RATES Perinatal[1]	6	19·9	24·8	18·8	16·8	22·7	25·0	21·8	21·5
Post-neonatal[2]	7	4·8	6·2	... 5·9	4·8	6·0	1·6	4·3	7·5
Infant[3]	8	14·4	19·3	15·5	16·5	18·6	14·3	16·7	18·7
1–4 years[4]	9	0·43	0·71	0·74	0·75	0·69	1·13	0·78	0·39
5–14 years[4]	10	0·36	0·32	0·39	0·21	0·28	0·20	0·26	0·36
0–14 years[4]	11	1·17	1·50	1·29	1·29	1·48	1·26	1·29	1·37
HEALTH SERVICES Hospital beds per 100,000 population 0–14 by specialty Paediatrics	12	76	50	53	91	77	—	171	141
Infectious diseases	13	51	14	25	8	41	—	13	45
Ear, nose and throat ...	14	53	93	49	32	50	1	100	86
Special care babies	15	48	15	54	42	26	—	39	39
Psychiatry	16	28	—	12	—	—	—	—	—
FAMILY PRACTITIONER COUNCILS Percentage of GPs[5] in Health Centres	17	6·2	16·3	16·6	5·6	30·5	51·7	23·8	31·3
Number of GPs[5] per 10,000 population 0–14	18	18·1	23·5	18·0	24·8	18·3	28·0	20·8	19·3
Average GP's[5] list size	19	2,322	2,051	2,318	1,797	2,370	1,870	2,112	2,303
Number of GDPs[6] per 10,000 population 0–14	20	6·0	8·1	7·5	9·1	6·2	7·9	10·7	8·9
COMMUNITY NURSES Home nurses per 10,000 population 0–14	21	12·4	20·0	13·8	15·7	10·8	18·6	10·1	13·0
Health visitors per 10,000 population 0–14	22	5·7	5·0	6·0	7·6	6·9	11·0	6·8	7·5
Midwives per 10,000 women 15–44	23	7·1	5·1	6·2	8·3	5·5	21·7	0·9	4·8
SCHOOL HEALTH SERVICE Nurses per 10,000 population 5–14	24	3·5	2·5	0·6	1·3	6·2	1·9	1·4	4·1

[1] Still births plus deaths of infants under one week per 1,000 live and still births.
[2] Deaths of infants aged 4 weeks and under one year per 1,000 live births.
[3] Deaths of infants under one year of age per 1,000 live births.
[4] Deaths per 1,000 population.
[5] General Medical Practitioners.
[6] General Dental Practitioners.

NOTE: It is necessary to be careful when comparing rates for AHAs as the provision of services may be changing rapidly over time.

Sources: Population statistics (item 1), live birth rates (item 5) and mortality rates (items 6–11) supplied by OPCS. Hospital services statistics (items 12–16) from the Welsh Office.

REGIONAL HOSPITAL BOARD AREAS ENGLAND AND WALES
1973

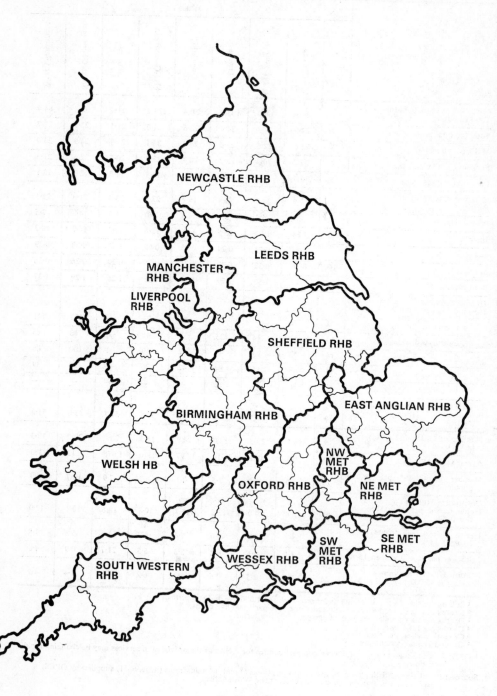

REGIONAL HEALTH AUTHORITY AREAS OF ENGLAND
(FROM 1 APRIL 1974)

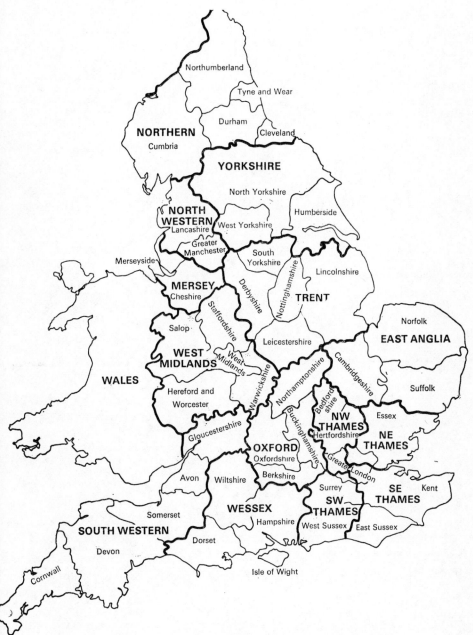

REGIONAL HEALTH AUTHORITY AREAS

Northern Region

The metropolitan county of Tyne and Wear and the non-metropolitan counties of Cleveland, Cumbria, Durham and Northumberland.

Yorkshire Region

The metropolitan county of West Yorkshire and the non-metropolitan counties of Humberside and North Yorkshire.

Trent Region

The metropolitan county of South Yorkshire and the non-metropolitan counties of Derbyshire, Leicestershire, Lincolnshire and Nottinghamshire.

East Anglian Region

The non-metropolitan counties of Cambridgeshire, Norfolk and Suffolk.

North West Thames Region

The non-metropolitan counties of Bedfordshire and Hertfordshire and the London boroughs of Barnet, Brent, Ealing, Hammersmith, Harrow, Hillingdon, Hounslow, Kensington and Chelsea, and Westminster.

North East Thames Region

The non-metropolitan county of Essex, the London boroughs of Barking, Camden, Enfield, Hackney, Haringey, Havering, Islington, Newham, Redbridge, Tower Hamlets and Waltham Forest, and the City of London.

South East Thames Region

The non-metropolitan counties of East Sussex and Kent and the London boroughs of Bexley, Bromley, Greenwich, Lambeth, Lewisham and Southwark.

South West Thames Region

The non-metropolitan counties of Surrey and West Sussex and the London boroughs of Croydon, Kingston-upon-Thames, Merton, Richmond-upon-Thames, Sutton and Wandsworth.

Wessex Region

The non-metropolitan counties of Dorset, Hampshire, Isle of Wight and Wiltshire.

Oxford Region

The non-metropolitan counties of Berkshire, Buckinghamshire, Northamptonshire and Oxfordshire.

South Western Region

The non-metropolitan counties of Avon, Cornwall, Devon, Gloucestershire and Somerset.

West Midlands Region

The metropolitan county of West Midlands and the non-metropolitan counties of Hereford and Worcester, Salop, Staffordshire and Warwickshire.

Mersey Region

The metropolitan county of Merseyside and the non-metropolitan county of Cheshire.

North Western Region

The metropolitan county of Greater Manchester and the non-metropolitan county of Lancashire.

REGIONAL HOSPITAL AREAS
ENGLAND

Newcastle Region

The administrative counties of Cumberland, Durham and Northumberland, the county boroughs of Carlisle, Darlington, Gateshead, Newcastle upon Tyne, South Shields, Sunderland, Teesside, Tynemouth and West Hartlepool.

So much of the administrative county of Westmorland as comprises the borough of Appleby and the rural district of North Westmorland. So much of the administrative county of the North Riding of York as comprises the borough of Richmond and the urban districts of Guisborough, Loftus, Northallerton, Saltburn and Marske-by-the-Sea, and Skelton and Brotton; and the rural districts of Croft, Northallerton, Reeth, Richmond, Startforth and Stokesley.

Leeds Region

The administrative counties of the East Riding of York, the North Riding of York (except the part included in the Newcastle Regional Hospital Area) and the West Riding of York (except the part included in the Sheffield Regional Hospital Area). The county boroughs of Bradford, Dewsbury, Halifax, Huddersfield, Kingston-upon-Hull, Leeds, Wakefield and York.

Sheffield Region

The administrative counties of Derby (except the part included in the Manchester Regional Hospital Area), Leicester, Lincoln, parts of Holland, Lincoln, parts of Kesteven (except the part included in the East Anglian Regional Hospital Area), Lincoln, parts of Lindsey, Nottingham and Rutland (except the rural district of Ketton). The county boroughs of Barnsley, Derby, Doncaster, Grimsby, Leicester, Lincoln, Nottingham, Rotherham and Sheffield.

So much of the administrative county of the West Riding of York as comprises the urban districts of Adwick-le-Street, Bentley with Arksey, Conisbrough, Cudworth, Darfield, Darton, Dearne, Dodworth, Hoyland Nether, Maltby, Mexborough, Penistone, Rawmarsh, Royston, Stocksbridge, Swinton,Tickhill, Wath-upon-Dearne, Wombwell and Worsborough; and the rural districts of Doncaster, Kiveton Park, Penistone, Rotherham, Thorne and Wortley.

East Anglian Region

The Counties of Cambridgeshire and Isle of Ely, Huntingdon andPeterborough, Norfolk, East Suffolk and West Suffolk.

The county boroughs of Great Yarmouth, Ipswich and Norwich.

In the county of Essex—the borough of Saffron Walden; the rural district of Saffron Walden.

In the county of Hertfordshire—the urban district of Royston.

In the county of Lincoln, parts of Kesteven—the borough of Stamford; the urban district of Bourne; the rural district of South Kesteven.

In the county of Rutland—the rural district of Ketton.

North-West Metropolitan Region

The counties of Bedford and Hertfordshire (except so much as is included in the East Anglian and North-East Metropolitan Regional Hospital Areas).

The county borough of Luton.

In the county of Surrey—the urban districts of Staines and Sunbury-on-Thames.

In the county of Berkshire—the boroughs of Maidenhead and New Windsor; the rural districts of Cookham, Easthampstead and Windsor.

In the county of Buckingham—the borough of Slough; the urban districts of Beaconsfield and Eton; the rural district of Eton.

In Greater London—the London boroughs of Barnet, Brent, Camden, Ealing, Harrow, Hillingdon, Hounslow and Islington; so much of the London borough of Haringey as lies west of Great Cambridge Road, the Roundway, Westbury Avenue and Green Lanes; so much of the London borough of Hammersmith as lies north of Goldhawk Road and Stamford Brook Road; so much of the Royal borough of Kensington and Chelsea as lies north of Holland Park Avenue, Notting Hill Gate and Bayswater Road; so much of the city of Westminster as lies north of Bayswater Road, north-east of Park Lane and north of Constitution Hill, Birdcage Walk, Great George Street, and Bridge Street; so much of the London borough of Enfield as is bounded by Blagdens Lane, High Street, The Meadway, Bourne Avenue, The Bourne, the boundary of Grovelands Hospital, Queen Elizabeth's Drive and the western end of The Bourne; and so much of the London borough of Richmond upon Thames as lies west of the River Thames.

North-East Metropolitan Region

The county of Essex (except so much as is included in the East Anglian Regional Hospital Area).

The county borough of Southend-on-Sea.

In the county of Hertfordshire—the borough of Hertford; the urban districts of Bishop's Stortford, Cheshunt, Hoddesdon, Sawbridgeworth and Ware; the rural districts of Braughing, Hertford and Ware.

In Greater London—the London boroughs of Barking, Hackney, Havering, Newham, Redbridge, Tower Hamlets and Waltham Forest; the London borough of Haringey (except so much as is included in the North-West Metropolitan Regional Hospital Area); the London borough of Enfield (except so much as is included in the North-West Metropolitan Regional Hospital Area); the City of London; and the Inner Temple and the Middle Temple.

South-East Metropolitan Region

The counties of Kent and East Sussex.

The county boroughs of Brighton, Canterbury, Eastbourne and Hastings.

In Greater London—the London boroughs of Bexley, Bromley, Greenwich and Lewisham; the whole of the London borough of Southwark (except the part lying west of Blackfriars Road, S.E.1, London Road, S.E.1 and Newington Butts, S.E.1, and S.E.11); and the part of the London borough of Lambeth lying east of the line Kennington Park Road, S.E.11, Brixton Road, S.W.9, Brixton Hill, S.W.2, Upper Tulse Hill, S.W.2, Roupell Road, S.W.2, Christ-church Road, S.W.2, Hillside Road, S.W.2, Palace Road, S.W.2, Kinfauns Road, S.W.2, Leigham Vale, S.W.2 and S.W.16, and Leigham Court Road, S.W.16.

South-West Metropolitan Region

The counties of Surrey (except so much as is included in the North-West Metropolitan Regional Hospital Area) and West Sussex.

In the county of Hampshire—the borough of Aldershot; the urban districts of Farnborough and Fleet; in the rural district of Hartley Wintney—the parishes of Yateley, Hawley, Crookham Village and Crondall (except enclosures Nos. 465, 467 to 470, 525, 526, 529, 530, 532 to 535 and 537 on the 1/2500 ordnance map of Hampshire (Sheets XXVIII, 2, 3, 6 and 7—1910 Edition)).

In Greater London—the London boroughs of Croydon, Kingston upon Thames, Merton, Sutton and Wandsworth; the London borough of Richmond upon Thames (except so much as is included in the North-West Metropolitan Regional Hospital Area); so much of the London borough of Hammersmith as lies south of Goldhawk Road and Stamford Brook Road; so much of the Royal borough of Kensington and Chelsea as lies south of Holland Park Avenue, Notting Hill Gate and Bayswater Road; so much of the city of Westminster as lies south of Bayswater Road, south-west of Park Lane and south of Constitution Hill, Birdcage Walk, Great George Street and Bridge Street; so much of the London borough of Lambeth as lies west of Kennington Park Road, Brixton Road and Brixton Hill, south-west of Upper Tulse Hill, west of Roupell Road, south of Christchurch Road, west of Hillside Road, south of Palace Road, west of Kinfauns Road and Leigham Vale and south and west of Leigham Court Road; and so much of the London borough of Southwark as lies west of Blackfriars Road, London Road and Newington Butts.

Wessex Region

The administrative counties of Dorset (except the part included in the South Western Regional Hospital Area), Isle of Wight and Hampshire (except the part included in the South-West Metropolitan Regional Hospital Area). The county boroughs of Bournemouth, Portsmouth and Southampton. So much of the administrative county of Wiltshire, as comprises the boroughs of New Sarum and Wilton; and the rural districts of Amesbury, Mere and Tisbury and Salisbury and Wilton.

Oxford Region

The counties of Berkshire (except so much as is included in the North-West Metropolitan Regional Hospital Area), Buckingham (except so much as is included in the North-West Metropolitan Regional Hospital Area), North-amptonshire and Oxford.

The county boroughs of Northampton, Oxford and Reading.

In the county of Gloucestershire—the urban district of Cirencester; the rural districts of Cirencester, North Cotswold and Northleach.

In the county of Wiltshire—the boroughs of Marlborough and Swindon; the rural districts of Cricklade and Wootton Bassett, Highworth, Marlborough and Ramsbury and Pewsey.

South Western Region

The administrative counties of Cornwall, Devon, Gloucester (excluding the urban district of Cirencester and the rural districts of Cirencester, North Cotswold and Northleach (Oxford Region)), Somerset and Wiltshire (except the parts included in the Wessex Regional Hospital Area and the Oxford Regional Hospital Area). The Isles of Scilly. The county boroughs of Bath, Bristol, Exeter, Gloucester and Plymouth.

So much of the administrative county of Dorset as comprises the borough of Lyme Regis.

Birmingham Region

The administrative counties of Hereford, Salop, Stafford, Warwick and Worcester. The county boroughs of Birmingham, Burton-upon-Trent, Coventry, Dudley, Solihull, Stoke-on-Trent, Walsall, Warley, West Bromwich, Wolverhampton and Worcester.

Manchester Region

The administrative counties of Chester (except the part included in the Liverpool Regional Hospital Area), Lancaster (except the part included in the Liverpool Regional Hospital Area) and Westmorland (except the part included in the Newcastle Regional Hospital Area). The county boroughs of Barrow-in-Furness, Blackburn, Blackpool, Bolton, Burnley, Bury, Manchester, Oldham, Preston, Rochdale, Salford, Stockport and Wigan.

So much of the county of Derby as comprises the boroughs of Buxton and Glossop; the urban districts of New Mills and Whaley Bridge; and the rural district of Chapel-en-le-Frith.

Liverpool Region

The county boroughs of Birkenhead, Bootle, Chester, Liverpool, St. Helens, Southport, Wallasey and Warrington.

So much of the administrative county of Chester as comprises the boroughs of Bebington and Ellesmere Port; the urban districts of Hoylake, Lymm, Neston, Runcorn and Wirral; the rural districts of Chester, Runcorn and Tarvin; and so much of the rural district of Northwich as comprises the parish of Tarporley. So much of the administrative county of Lancaster as comprises the boroughs of Crosby and Widnes; the urban districts of Formby, Golborne, Haydock, Huyton with Roby, Litherland, Newton-le-Willows, Ormskirk, Prescot, Rainford and Skelmersdale New Town; and the rural districts of Warrington, West Lancashire and Whiston.

WALES

Welsh Hospital Area

The whole of Wales and the administrative county of Monmouth. The county borough of Newport.

Printed in England for Her Majesty's Stationery Office by Oyez Press Limited
Dd. 294753 K60 12/76